YOU'VE GOT THIS

You've Got This

Seven Steps to a Life You Love

DR MICHAELA DUNBAR

MICHAEL JOSEPH

PENGUIN MICHAEL JOSEPH

of companies
.com

First published 2022

001

Copyright © Dr Michaela Dunbar, 2022

The moral right of the author has been asserted

Page 112, copyright © Dr Russ Harris, *ACT for Worrying, Ruminating & Obsessing* (July 29, 2021)

Every effort has been made to trace copyright holders and to obtain their permission for the use of copyright material. The publisher apologizes for any errors or omissions and would be grateful to be notified of any corrections that should be incorporated in future editions of this book.

Set in 13.12/15.49pt Garamond MT Std
Typeset by Jouve (UK), Milton Keynes
Printed and bound in Great Britain by Clays Ltd, Elcograf S.p.A.

The authorized representative in the EEA is Penguin Random House Ireland,
Morrison Chambers, 32 Nassau Street, Dublin D02 YH68

A CIP catalogue record for this book is available from the British Library

ISBN: 978-0-241-54574-4

www.greenpenguin.co.uk

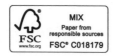

To every girl who ever doubted herself.
Trust me, you've got this.
Love, Michaela x

Contents

trust me, you've got this

INTRODUCTION

Let me be honest with you, psychology is a career I kind of fell into.

For a long time I didn't even know clinical psychology was a real job – I thought it was just something you saw on TV dramas. And it certainly wasn't the sort of thing a girl from rowdy Lewisham would grow up thinking was an option for her. At my school, if you left without a baby, that was considered a win.

But here we are!

I was a low-key nerd at school. I wasn't academic, but I worked hard, kept out of trouble and, as a result, I managed to get an undergraduate degree. I chose to study psychology purely because I'd quite enjoyed it at A level and didn't really know what else to do.

I ended up falling hook, line and sinker for it. The more I learned, the more fascinated I became, and by the time I got accepted on to my doctorate I knew there was nothing else I would rather be doing with my life.

A major reason for that was wanting to help empower women to unlock their full potential. I worked across lots of different client groups during my research roles and placements, but it was with them that I always got my best results. I felt most energetic and passionate working with women.

The women I was seeing were ambitious and driven but trapped by anxiety, overthinking, imposter syndrome and a crippling fear of failure. And so lacking in confidence that they were probably giving only 55 per cent of themselves.

We know that women are already at structural and systemic disadvantages as soon as they step into the workplace, and here was a whole group of people whose talents were being stifled even further by their own difficult emotions and intrusive thoughts. They were successful in their fields and working on huge projects with global brands – I could clearly see how brilliant and bright they were. I just needed them to join the dots and believe it themselves.

As someone who had spent her whole life wrestling with anxiety and doubt, I knew how they were feeling. I am unapologetically myself today, but it took time to get to this point. I am a wounded healer who is not above struggle, and I'm going to share with you more about my journey throughout this book.

Before we go any further, you should know that my style of therapy is different to a lot of the prescriptive psychology out there. I like to cut through the bullshit, and I'm not a fan of jargon. I don't have a therapy voice. You know, all softly spoken and head-tilty. My sessions are a mix of fun and serious. We can joke – not everything has to be heavy!

Sure, I use the trusted and established models, but I also need to connect with people, validate them and show empathy, and leaving the NHS to set up my own private practice has given me more freedom to do things my way.

In this book we're going to talk about stuff that is hard, but I'm going to give it a lighter flavour. This is an easy introduction to sorting out your mental wellbeing, and I hope we can also chip away at some of the stigma that still exists around seeking therapy or admitting we need help.

For some reason, even now, there's shame in saying: 'I'm not OK, I feel shit,' or 'I cried for an hour last night and woke up feeling worse.' Instead, we tend to say: 'Yeah, I'm good, thanks. How are you?' with a smile, regardless of the turmoil going on beneath that brave face.

I used to be a hundred per cent guilty of this. You'd never catch me telling people my problems – I was the therapist, after all! I finally managed to break what Dr Russ Harris calls 'the conspiracy of silence', except I started by sharing my thoughts with a few hundred thousand Instagram followers ... and *then* I made my way back to my real-life bestie and told her too!

The result of this was both overwhelming and under-whelming for me. On the one hand, I felt good. But when the judgement I'd feared from others, which for years had stopped me speaking up, never actually came and I was just left feeling better ... how anticlimactic for my cata-strophic and melodramatic thoughts was that?!

Since launching @MyEasyTherapy in October 2019, we've created a lovely (not so) little community where people share their experiences and help each other. I can hardly believe there are so many of us – more than 700,000 – but it feels really cool to be a part of it.

So, that's me. How about you? Do you feel good enough to be able to get through the issues that are holding you back? If the answer is currently no, we're going to get you to yes. This will work for you. It's hard but, you know what? It's not *that* hard. It's doable.

The thing you think is unique to you and makes you somehow defective? No. This is a human being issue, not a you issue. And if you take on board what we're going to explore together, there is no way you won't see a change by the end of it.

Each one of these chapters is about setting the foundations for anything in life you want to go on to do next. They will give you the basics that will keep you afloat, hopefully for ever.

I want you to promise me one thing though: that you won't let this book gather dust on the shelf (it's too cute for that). Read it, implement these practices and you will become a person who can have any thought, and any feeling, and still do what the f*** she needs to do to get to where she needs to be.

You deserve this, and I'm excited for you because I can totally see what's in there. Just remember, I'm here, right behind you all the way. So let's do it together.

Trust me, you've got this.

CHAPTER ONE

The Five-Part Model

'Watch your thoughts, they become words;
watch your words, they become actions;
watch your actions, they become habits;
watch your habits, they become character.'

– Lao Tzu

trying to control
our emotions is
like trying to
control the weather:

IT JUST
AIN'T
GONNA
HAPPEN

So, I'm guessing you're feeling pretty stuck in some areas of your life right now. First things first: what you're experiencing at this moment is temporary. And, honestly, it's always been temporary – you just didn't know it. Why is that important? Well, if you knew that the overthinking, the desire to people-please, and the feelings of high anxiety and imposter syndrome had an end point, would you feel differently about them? I suspect you would.

Knowing we have a pathway out of a bad situation solves half of the problem. The second half is solved by walking down it. This chapter is going to get you ready for that pathway, and then the rest of the book will take you along it and out the other side.

I'm a problem-solver. I always have been, and I always will be. Yes, I'm a clinical psychologist, but I see myself as more of an empathetic mind detective. People come to me with problems, stuck in a tangled web of difficult emotions, negative thoughts and unhelpful behaviours. I help them to separate out the various parts of this web and figure out what stays, what goes and what we need to add in order for them to feel in control of their emotions and live their lives in the way they want to.

Let's break it down

I get it. Sometimes when you're dealing with problems (aka the shit that life throws at you) it can feel totally over-whelming and you don't know where to start. When you're in this situation, I find it's helpful to break a problem down using Padesky's Five-part Model (no need to reinvent the wheel, right?).

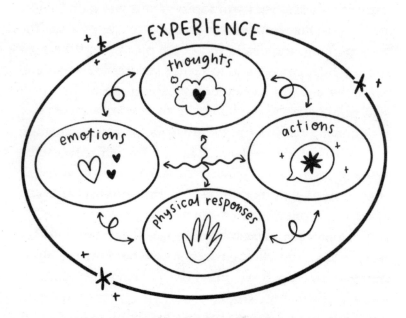

Each of these parts interacts with the others for good, or for evil . . . just kidding! I'm being dramatic here. What

I mean is, one small change in each individual area can lead to big changes in another, and the positive knock-on effects just keep going.

We're going to start by mapping out these five parts for you and looking at what emotions, thoughts, physical responses, actions and experiences make up your vicious cycle. Having a deeper understanding of each of the parts will mean it's much easier to identify the areas you need to change.

REFLECTION EXERCISE

There are going to be a few of these, so grab a notebook and sit down with a cuppa! Write down answers to the following:

Emotions
What single words describe my most frequent or troubling moods – sad, nervous, angry, guilty, ashamed?

Thoughts
When I have strong moods, what thoughts do I have about myself, other people, my future? What sort of thoughts interfere with me doing the things I'd like to do or that I think I should do? What images or memories come into my mind?

Physical responses
What physical symptoms am I having? Think energy levels, appetite, pain and sleep as well as occasional symptoms

such as muscle tension, tiredness, rapid heartbeat, stomach aches, sweating, dizziness and breathing difficulties.

Actions

What behaviours are connected to my moods? Behaviours are the things that we do or avoid doing. Think about how your behaviours manifest themselves at work, at home, with friends or when you're by yourself, because of how you're feeling.

Experiences

What recent changes have there been in my life – positive as well as negative? What have been the most stressful events for me in the past year? Three years? Five years? In childhood? Am I experiencing any long-term ongoing challenges?

OK, what did you notice from that exercise? Your thoughts and moods are totally connected, right? And you might also have noticed that your previous experiences have had an impact on your behaviour today and that your behaviour today is very changeable depending on what mood you are in.

That, my friend, is being human.

Now, if the connections you can see are all doom and gloom and leave you feeling hopeless in this vicious cycle, bear with me, because the good news is that we can make tiny positive changes to turn this whole vicious cycle into a virtuous cycle. I know that sounds super-cheesy, but I honestly didn't make that up – that's legit psychology speak!

Throughout this book, we're going to identify your exit points from this vicious cycle, then guide you towards them, and through them.

* we can make tiny, positive *
changes to turn this whole +
+ + vicious cycle into a +
* + = virtuous cycle. = *

It wasn't so long ago that I was in your shoes. I spent my whole life feeling like I wasn't good enough and that I didn't fit in. I worried about what other people thought of me, always terrified of being judged or disliked and, ultimately, rejected. This followed me from primary school, where I became super-competitive due to the fear of how my eight-year-old friends would judge me if I wasn't a genius in maths (yes, my school was strange), to high school, when my parents were called in within months of me being there because, although I was intelligent and loved learning, I started hanging around with 'the wrong crowd', pretended I didn't like studying and acted very unlike myself as I tried to fit in (this would become a theme). Did it stop there? Of course not. Fast-forward to 2019, and I'm in my early thirties, working as a clinical psychologist in the NHS and diving headfirst into burn-out.

Let me set the scene. I had been working in my service for a few years. Killing it. I can say that confidently now. As time went on, government funding started to get tighter and tighter, the interest in mental health services seemed to get smaller and smaller, and as a result the waiting lists became longer and longer – and this was the case even before the pandemic.

I was working like a machine, seeing patients back to back, giving myself little down time, saying, 'Yes, of course I'll be involved,' to any new initiatives my senior colleagues thought up to try and tackle the problems that, in my opinion, the people who were running the country had created. People always say that psychologists shouldn't talk about politics, but I don't care; it's so intertwined it's impossible not to. Anyway, yes, we were understaffed and underfunded, like most mental health services in the UK, but if I'm completely honest, it was my own 'stuff' that was keeping me stuck. My unhelpful thoughts, my self-doubt and my fear of abandonment. Deep, right? I liked being the one who people trusted to come in and save the day. I liked feeling needed. I believed that gave me value in the team, and that made me feel safe. I was scared of what might happen if I started to put in boundaries. This fuelled me to say yes when I knew I should have screamed, 'Hell, no!'

I loved the client work and gave a hundred per cent in every session I did, but otherwise my energy levels were zero, my stomach was in bits, my childhood migraines re-started and both my internal and my external world were becoming unbearable. My usual positive outlook had diminished and I just couldn't get started with work. Normally, it would just be the boring bits I'd procrastinate on, but now I didn't have the motivation to do anything. I'd wake up every morning and have about one and a half seconds of calm before the anxiety kicked in. It was like clockwork. I went from being enthusiastic and playful to being cynical and irritable. I felt trapped, and I was ready to pack it all in and become a florist. But I didn't, I stayed, because I didn't want to let the team, who I genuinely loved and respected, down – and I stayed too long. By the time I did leave I had felt so unhappy and so unlike myself for such a long time it was an easy decision to go.

It was a long way back from being emotionally and physically burnt out, and, by the grace of God, I did make it back. (You might think being religious wouldn't mesh with being a 'scientist-practitioner', but it works for me.) And now that I've got a handle on the techniques we're going to discuss in this book, I have all the tools I need to work through any unhelpful thoughts that pop into my head and threaten to derail my actions and my day. I honour my emotions instead of running from them and making things worse, and everything I do has my values of self-love, compassion and boundaries at the centre.

My starting point for getting to where I am now was applying the Five-part Model to myself. Don't assume that therapists have their shit together. We mostly don't, but we're really good at helping everyone else get their shit together. Understanding the Five-part Model is going to change everything for you, but first let's take a look at each section and bust some of the myths. There are many.

Emotions

Myth: People should be happy all the time, and if you aren't, there's something wrong with you.

Truth: Emotions are like knickers – expect them to change all the time.

If your goal is to be happy all the time, then I'm gonna have to stop you right there and let you know that's not realistic. Every single emotion you have the ability to feel is necessary, and each one serves an important function. Yes, some can feel crippling at times, but sometimes they have to feel awful so that you address them.

Can you imagine if we never felt fear? If that car coming towards us at full speed didn't faze us, it would just run us over. As I said, some emotions need to feel bad enough for us to pay attention to them and act to change the situation.

Difficult emotions are not something that we should aspire to avoid. We should learn how to manage them, and manage them well. A key thing to remember is that emotions are going to manifest differently depending on the person in the situation. Some of the ways we show our emotions are hardwired into us, and it's pretty much going to look the same whoever you are. It's natural for us to cry when we feel sad and give an Angry Bird face when we're furious.

What's different between us is our *experience* of an emotion, and that's because it's not just a feeling, it's accompanied by so many different thoughts, urges and physiological sensations. And there are so many different factors that influence how an emotion feels for someone.

Factors such as the people involved, what space you are in and what circumstances are looming over you.

Myth: You can control your emotions.
Truth: Trying to control your emotions is like trying to control the weather – it just ain't gonna happen.

If you're alive, you're going to experience difficult emotions. It's just part of being human. Trying to control our emotions usually takes us away from showing up in the way we want to, from engaging with people and living in line with what's truly meaningful to us.

You can't just turn your emotions on and off at will, but there's a reason we believe we can and it lies with the adults we had around us growing up. They, through no fault of their own, subconsciously gave us the message that it was possible to control our emotions, with 'helpful' comments such as 'Don't cry,' 'Don't be a scaredy-cat,' 'Stop feeling sorry for yourself.' Then we went to school and heard the same thing from the other kids, who had been told all that, too.

None of that is healthy emotion regulation, but let's be clear, there's no judgement of our parents here. As with everything in this book, judgement is off the table. There's no such thing as Parent School, and they likely went through exactly the same things with their own parents.

Most of us try to escape any feeling that is not 'happy' or 'calm' or that just doesn't feel good. And the strategies we use to escape them usually end up backfiring. We might try to suppress our feelings by forcing ourselves not to think about that 'thing' because it makes us feel unhappy.

Or we might enrol our internal frenemy to shout at us: 'You're such a cry-baby! Why do you even care that he's with Lauren now? You were never official anyway!'

If we're in a situation which isn't that stressful or important, and the feelings aren't that intense, it will be easier to make an intentional shift in our emotional state. You might procrastinate to put off feeling the inevitable boredom while writing that proposal, or you might cancel that work dinner because Annie from accounts is going to be there and she's mean and well put together and she makes you feel anxious, and obviously you'll probably end up seated next to her . . .

But try using those avoidance techniques when you're waiting for MRI scan results or breaking up with your partner. I mean . . . no, they just won't work. That anxiety isn't going anywhere.

REFLECTION EXERCISE

For the next week, I want you to notice all the things you do every day to avoid unwanted thoughts and feelings. Note down the consequences of these behaviours: what did you do? How did it make you feel?

The faster you notice that these behaviours aren't helping you and that you're stuck in a trap, the faster you can lift yourself out of it.

Thoughts

Myth: Thoughts are facts.
Truth: Thoughts are more like well-curated stories.

And with any type of story, some will have evidence that backs up the detail, and others won't. However, we still react to them as if they're the absolute truth because the mind is a great storyteller. Think about all the stories your mind has told you today: 'I should've done that extra piece of work,' 'I'm not good enough for that job,' 'I'll never be able to get all that washing done.'

Our minds never stop telling stories, and the difficult thing is that our minds evolved to think negatively – research suggests that 80 per cent of our thoughts have some degree of negative content. Now, these thoughts aren't a problem if we see them as they are – merely words in our minds – but when we 'fuse' with them they can become problematic, feeding into our emotions and behaviour.

I'm going to tell you a quick story to really hammer home my point. This morning, I really fancied a strong coffee. I took a cold, smooth spoon from the drawer and ground it into my jar of instant, feeling the sensation as the granules crumbled underneath it. I brought the spoon to my nose and took a moment to smell the coffee before putting it into the cup. As I poured over the boiling water, I watched as the granules melted away and I added a splash of creamy oat milk before bringing the cup to my nose again for another long inhale of the warm, coffee-scented air. I held the cup in both hands, feeling its warmth, and took a sip.

Did anything happen as you read my little anecdote? Did you picture it in your mind and imagine the warmth of the cup and the smell of the coffee? Did you end up fancying a coffee afterwards? Or maybe you hate coffee and started to feel nauseous? Sorry!

But this is how powerful your mind can be – there might be no coffee in front of you, only words describing it, yet you reacted to them almost as if you had a cup too. The same things happen when you watch a scary movie or hear about something awful on the news.

Now imagine the words in your mind were negative and critical about yourself. You're fat, you're lazy, you're never going to get that promotion, you're going to fail. What feelings would that stir up in you? Would you feel happy, peaceful or content?

Chances are, you would feel the complete opposite to that because – you got it – our thoughts heavily influence our emotions. Most of the time it doesn't matter if the thought is true. What matters is whether fusing with it is helpful or not. Is aligning yourself with this thought or way of thinking going to take you in the direction you want to go, or need to go? Or will it encourage you to show up in the way you want to? Does it motivate you and guide you in the direction of the kind of life you want? If not, then, frankly, it doesn't need your attention.

This book is going to arm you with the skills you need to turn your attention away from these thoughts and enable you to get on with things that are much more meaningful.

Myth: We can suppress negative thoughts.
Truth: Trying to suppress thoughts will make them come knocking on your door harder than your ex after a drunken night out.

trying to SUPPRESS thoughts, will make them come knocking on your door HARDER than your ex after a drunken night out! (HeLLO?)

Numerous studies have shown that trying to suppress thoughts increases the likelihood they will come back – a phenomenon known as the 'rebound effect'. And it's now believed that thought suppression has an impact on your behaviour.

In a study by social psychologist Daniel Wegner in 1998, participants were asked to try to suppress the urge to move a pendulum in a certain direction. The result? Yep, they all ended up moving the pendulum in that exact direction.

Participants who were given a simultaneous mental load (in this case, initially, having to count backwards from 1,000 in threes) were told to suppress thoughts of over-putting a golf ball – and what do you reckon happened? Correct – they ended up over-putting the golf ball even more frequently.

Basically, thought suppression is a battle and it's one that can't be won but takes up a lot of time and energy when we attempt to do it. Come on, we've all experienced that feeling when we actively try to avoid certain thoughts but instead find we're thinking about them even more, haven't we? Ultimately, you can't control your thoughts, so the most positive move you can make in this situation is to combine acceptance and action.

You don't have to like uncomfortable thoughts, or want them, or approve of them. You simply make peace with them and let them be. Remind yourself that you can't stop these thoughts from coming. The only thing you can control is how you react to them. Try to observe these thoughts coming in, accept them and move on. This leaves you free to focus your energy on taking action that moves you forward in a direction you value.

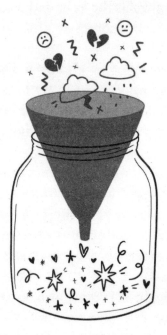

This is a good point to introduce you to negative mental filtering, which is when we only acknowledge things that fit with our negative core beliefs, ignoring any other input.

Think of it like a broken funnel that only lets through stuff which fits in with our negative thoughts and filters everything else out – including all the helpful contradictory stuff.

For example, you feel insecure about your likeability and every time a friend is late to call you back or seems preoccupied, it reaffirms your belief that people dislike you. You completely disregard any of the times when they act kindly towards you, as it doesn't fit the view that you have about yourself.

REFLECTION EXERCISE

If you find yourself in a similar situation take a step back and look at it through a different lens; see if you can identify any other detail in the situation that doesn't fit the same type of narrative that your mental filter usually lets through. Are there any anomalies that your mental filter left out?

Physical responses

Myth: You can't teach an old dog new tricks.
Truth: Neuroplasticity means that throughout our entire lives our brain is able to reorganize itself and form new neural pathways based on new things it learns.

The more you practise anything, the better you get. If you're practising judgement, impatience and frustration, those are the feelings that will grow. This isn't a theoretical woo-woo thing, this is a neuroscience thing – what we practise moment by moment physically alters our brain.

It's not just about what we pay attention to, it's how we

pay attention to it. If we're paying attention to something with judgement, we are literally growing judgement. I liken pruning flowers and plants to pruning our brains – we can trim away unhealthy pathways and, in the process, allow space to create new ones. That is neuroplasticity. And the best part is that we can do this at any point in our lives – age isn't a factor.

we can prune away UNHEALTHY pathways &, in the process, allow SPACE to create new ones. THAT IS NEUROPLASTICITY.

So we have endless potential here. If something serves you, you can strengthen it. If it doesn't, you can get rid of it. If you need something new, you can create it. How amazing is that? What's even more amazing is that you are about to do it. Your potential is literally limitless – you just need to pair intention with action.

I want you to become intentional about as many things in your life as you can. You're planting seeds unconsciously with every thought you give your attention to and every action you take. These seeds can turn into anything.

Let's make sure they turn into something beautiful.

Myth: Your gut has no impact on your mood – it's just marketing.
Truth: The mind/body connection is real. Believe the hype.

You've probably seen adverts pushing probiotic yoghurts to create a happy, smiling you and raised a cynical eyebrow. But the gut *can* have an impact on mental as well as physical health. In addition to being responsible for letting nutrients into the body, the gut microbiome – the trillions of micro-organisms living in your intestines – is also directly connected to the brain, along what is known as the gut–brain axis. Beware: science-nerd info loading.

So, how does this all work? Well, we do a lot of things necessary for survival without even thinking about it, like breathing, swallowing and digesting food. The vagus nerve – which connects the digestive organs to the brain – plays an important role in the gut–brain axis. When we're under stress, the vagus nerve gets inhibited and stops being able to control what toxins and bacteria can pass into the body and through to the brain.

This has a domino effect, impacting the gut–brain communication system, including the part of the brain that coordinates the 'fight or flight' response (which we'll talk a lot more about in Chapter 3, on anxiety).

Imagine coming home to find a strange man standing in your living room. The logical thing to do would be to get out as quickly as possible and, under these stressful situations, your body releases hormones such as adrenaline that shut down non-essential activities like digestion (which makes sense, since a full stomach could slow down your escape from this intruder), while activating muscles so they have more energy when escaping the imminent danger.

Now, finding an intruder in your living room is an extreme and very unlikely situation, but these same processes happen when we're feeling anxious after sending a risky text to Paul in PR. With these shutdowns come changes within the gut microbiome, too, and an unbalanced gut microbiome (scientists call that dysbiosis) can have a terrible impact on your mood, increasing anxiety levels and reducing stress resilience. There's also evidence to suggest it can exacerbate symptoms of depression.

In a nutshell, having more calm and balance in your gut means more calm and balance for your mental health, and the addition of probiotics into your diet and introducing other simple additions such as fibres found in whole foods like fruit and veg can have a beneficial impact on your mood.

So there's another good reason to add more plant-based food to your daily diet.

Actions

Myth: Emotions control our behaviour.
Truth: Behaviour is not controlled by anything except our intention.

We've talked about a lot of things that we can't control – our thoughts (don't even bother), our emotions (good luck with that) – but if there is one thing we *can* control, it's our actions. Our thoughts, emotions and actions – or behaviours – are all closely connected.

. BEHAVIOUR is not controlled .
by anything except our intention. +

Dr Russ Harris separates specific behaviours aimed at avoiding or suppressing – essentially controlling – uncomfortable thoughts and feelings as follows:

- Hiding
- Distraction
- Zoning out/numbing
- Suppression
- Arguing
- Taking charge
- Self-bullying

Recognize any of these? It's OK to do these things in moderation – and sometimes they do help you to get the courage and focus you need to move through tricky situations – but when you use them excessively, they can start to impact you negatively, and then you have a problem.

In the same way, even what we consider positive behaviours can end up being unhelpful. Something may *seem* positive, like giving to charity, joining a club or working out, but if you're only doing this to get rid of unpleasant thoughts and feelings in the process (hello, guilt), the chances are these actions won't be rewarding as you thought.

Myth: We don't have a choice in how we act.
Truth: Sorry, love, but nine times out of ten, how you show up is your choice (no judgement).

Good news is, with awareness and practice, we can make better choices. We do a lot each day, we make decisions, get jobs done and communicate with others. If you think about it, how many actions have you done today? How many of those actions took you towards the type of life you want? And how many took you away from it?

We can categorize these simply as Away moves and Towards moves. It's easy to take Towards moves when you're feeling good, but when you get sucked in by negative critical thoughts and the struggle to get rid of uncomfortable emotions, the Away moves are inevitable and the easiest course.

But the better we get at unhooking ourselves from these thoughts and feelings, the easier it is to make Towards moves that can get us on that path to what we want.

- Identify what drives and inspires you – your core values.
- Deal with any barriers, thoughts and feelings to making those Towards moves.

REFLECTION EXERCISE

Remind yourself of your goals by asking yourself the following questions:

What do you want to grow?
Where do you want to go?
Are the actions you're currently taking setting you up for success?
Or are they simply leading you to anxiety, procrastination, people-pleasing and worry?

Now connect with your goals and values and schedule a reminder on your phone every day of what these are to reinforce what you are trying to achieve.

Experience

Myth: If you don't meet the criteria for Post Traumatic Stress Disorder (PTSD), you haven't experienced trauma. **Truth:** Any event or series of events that a person found highly stressful has the ability to cause psychological trauma.

It's commonly known that having a near-death experience, living through war, sexual assault or any experience where you felt under threat or frightened can have a really damaging impact on our psychological wellbeing. Many of you reading this might be thinking, 'Well, I haven't had anything major happen to me, so why do I feel so bad?' Well, what's less commonly known is that childhood experiences that left you feeling abandoned, rejected, humiliated, unsupported or ashamed – for example, having a super-busy, well-meaning but unavailable parent, being constantly compared to your more 'able' sibling or being bullied at school can be experienced as traumatic and have lasting effects into adulthood.

Our environment and life experiences shape our beliefs and, in turn, the emotions and actions that dictate our lives. Single traumatic events can influence beliefs, but any part of your environment can influence the core beliefs you have about yourself today – it could be your family, your teachers, your community, where you live, your interactions with other people, your culture. You can be influenced by present and past experiences from your childhood to this moment. We'll be discussing different trauma responses throughout the book.

A dysfunctional environment keeps you in threat mode, so it's important to problem-solve and manage that environment, and making those changes can also help you feel better. Here are a few examples of what those changes might look like:

Saying no to unreasonable demands from people or
    things you just really don't want to do.
Spending more time with people who make you
    feel good.
Taking action to reduce discrimination at work.

Of course, with some situations, it's not enough just to change the way you think about it or manage your emotions in relation to that situation. Sometimes you need to take immediate action, for example where there are safety issues or abuse. Everything in this book is written with my readers' potential traumas in mind . . . I've got you.

Core beliefs

You might notice that there are times when it's hard to believe anything positive about yourself and the unhelpful critical thoughts seem to be very powerful. You might notice that this only happens in particular kinds of

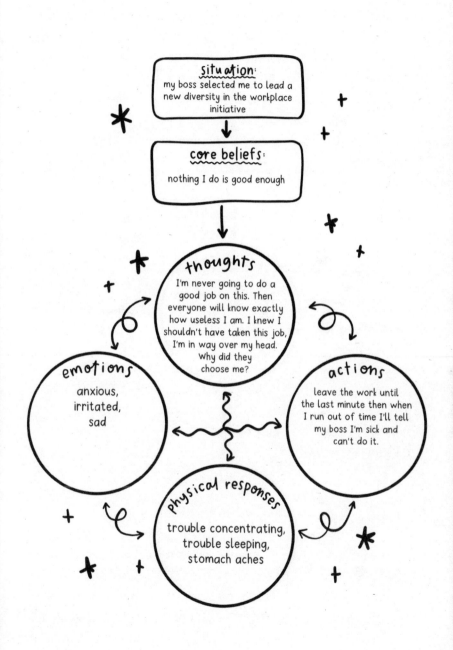

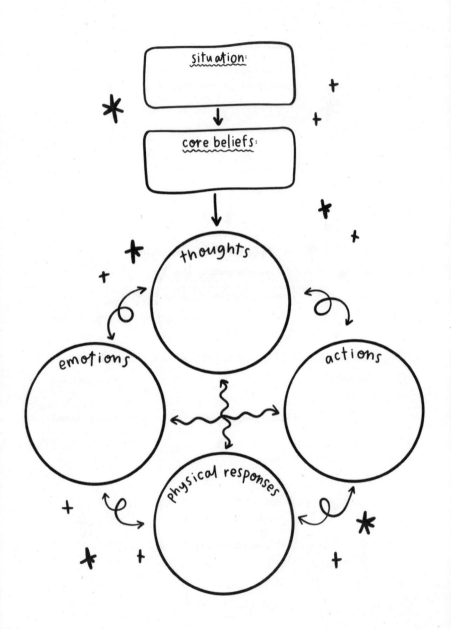

situations. One possible explanation for this difficulty in letting go of such thoughts is that there may be a strong core belief at the root of it.

Core beliefs are the very essence of how we see ourselves, other people, the world and the future. Sometimes, in certain situations, these core beliefs become 'activated'.

✳ ⹀CASE STUDY⹀ ✦

Anna is able to challenge her self-critical thinking in most situations. An unhelpful critical thought will come up, for example, 'You look awful today,' and she will be able to put it to the side and get on with her day.

However, she notices that she has trouble challenging her thinking in situations involving her colleagues. In these situations, she has recognized that her thinking is often about being unlikeable. In fact, when she really looks hard at her thinking, she can see that often the underlying self-statement is actually 'I'm unlovable.'

Core beliefs like Anna's develop over time, usually from childhood, from the experience of significant life events or tricky life circumstances. They are maintained by the tendency to focus on information that supports the belief and ignoring the evidence that contradicts it.

For example, Anna focuses on any feedback from her colleagues that isn't positive and then uses this to confirm she is unlikeable. Even neutral statements from her colleagues are often interpreted as negative. Over the years, this narrow focus gives strength to the belief, and Anna no longer thinks even to question it. It's just totally and absolutely accepted. This is why these types of beliefs are the hardest to shake.

While the majority of issues with sense of self can be traced back to early childhood or adolescence, there are experiences that can lower your sense of self as an adult. Traumatic experiences, consistent negativity, bullying or intimidation in the workplace and other similar factors can all chip away at what was an otherwise positive self-image. And especially if you're a deep-thinking and deep-feeling highly sensitive person (I'm going to explain *so* much more about HSPs in the next chapter), as these experiences will be processed differently and can be internalized to a different level.

Of course, negativity can't always be avoided, and nor should it be. But it's important to understand the impact that ongoing negativity can have on us. You're probably wondering how all these events, experiences and past happenings can linger for so long and affect us so far into the future. Why don't our adult experiences override those from early childhood?

Well, even with all this new information informing our world view, we may still hear our inner child telling us we are 'not good enough' or directing the same sorts of criticisms at ourselves that we have heard since we were young. This is the negative core belief system. For example, a child who was often punished or criticized develops into an adult who has feelings of worthlessness or fear. These feelings, and the ideas of self-worth they represent, are the negative core beliefs.

As a child, it's hard to know why the people around you act like they do, so you end up making up your own ideas about why they are treating you this way and you can end up internalizing their behaviour as something that's wrong with you. These ideas make sense to us as children – they allow us to understand in a simple way why we are being punished or criticized.

Unfortunately, during such a formative time in our lives, these thoughts can very quickly become foundational. And they turn into evaluations of ourselves that can last a lifetime if we aren't intentional about changing them.

Negative core beliefs can look like: 'I am unworthy,' 'I am ugly,' 'I am unintelligent,' 'I'll never succeed,' 'I'm a terrible person,' and so on. For you, your negative core beliefs may be difficult to specify or identify exactly. Because they often form so early in life, we may forget where they came from or be completely unaware of their origins.

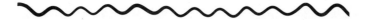

If you want to uncover your own core beliefs, create a timeline of all the difficult experiences you've had from as far back as you can remember. Reflect on these experiences in your life, if they are not too painful, and ask yourself this question: *Did this experience or experiences lead me to believe anything about myself? If so, was it negative?*

I know it may be tempting to think you don't have to write it down, that you can just remember the answers to these questions and think them through in your mind – I've been there. But I urge you to grab your notebook and write down your responses. Research shows that writing things down not only increases the chance of retaining the information but also helps you process and understand the information.

This can be a difficult exercise to do, so have someone with you if you need to, and if you have a therapist, perhaps do it with them. In any event, be sure to be kind to yourself during the process.

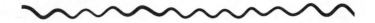

When we're overcome by our negative thoughts and feelings, it's so hard to show up as the best version of ourselves, and we slip into the default, which could look like people-pleasing, snapping at others, being vacant, not being present around our partners, and so on.

It's even harder when we don't actually know how we *want* to show up. I always ask my clients if unhelpful thoughts and uncomfortable emotions were not an issue for them, what would they be doing, how would they behave? This question is usually answered by: 'I really don't know, I can't imagine it . . . It's been this way for so long.'

If you're feeling the same, that's OK. Trust that if you are intentional about doing the work in this book, you are well on your way to becoming the person you want to be, whatever that looks like. The first step is getting a good understanding of what's important and meaningful to you. Deep in your heart, what do you want your life to be about? What do you want to stand for? What do you want to do with your brief time on this planet? What truly matters to you in the big picture? Just like earlier, this is a write-it-down kind of task and doing so is a sure-fire way to maximize change.

What are your values?

Values are desired qualities of ongoing action. In other words, they describe how we want to behave on an ongoing basis. Clarifying our values is an essential step in creating a meaningful life. I like to compare values to a compass, because they give us direction around how to show up in any given situation. They are leading principles that guide us and motivate us as we move through this tricky life.

Goals are great, but they can be broken or lost. Values are ongoing and consistent. If you wake up one day and you're not that person, it doesn't matter, there's always tomorrow. Even the next hour, you can get back on it.

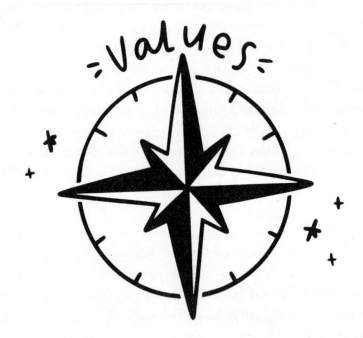

REFLECTION EXERCISE

Let's imagine it's your eightieth birthday, you're on a swanky yacht somewhere on the Med and all the guests are dressed up to the nines. Everyone from your past and your present, dead or alive, is here.

One by one, they stand up and say something about you. A parent, a sibling, an old colleague, your best friend. What would you hope they say? Do they say you're kind? Principled? Loyal? Creative? Ambitious?

The answers are what will form your values – the things you believe are important for how you live and work – and they are what should determine your priorities. Let them be your compass point.

Putting it into practice

Now you're familiar with the Five-part Model made up of emotions, thoughts, physical responses, actions and experiences and how they all interconnect, it will help you to assess your current life situation, define the areas where you need support and readjust your thinking to get the outcomes you want. We're all looking for happiness and contentment in our lives, and to achieve this we need to keep our mental health in balance as much as our crazy lifestyles. We should aspire to live a rich and meaningful life where we feel the full range of emotions without a struggle.

Most of us are good at the feel-good emotions, but now, hopefully, you understand that it's important that we feel *all* of them – comfortable and not so comfortable. The truth is, life involves pain, and we will all feel it, but I'm hoping this book will help you to handle these moments much better and use them to drive you forward to the life you want instead of making it harder by trying to avoid them.

Stick with me, and I will help you identify what you're feeling, understand what's causing those feelings and gather the skills you need to manage them so day-to-day living becomes a whole lot less stressful.

CHAPTER TWO

Highly Sensitive People

'My sensitivity is my superpower.'

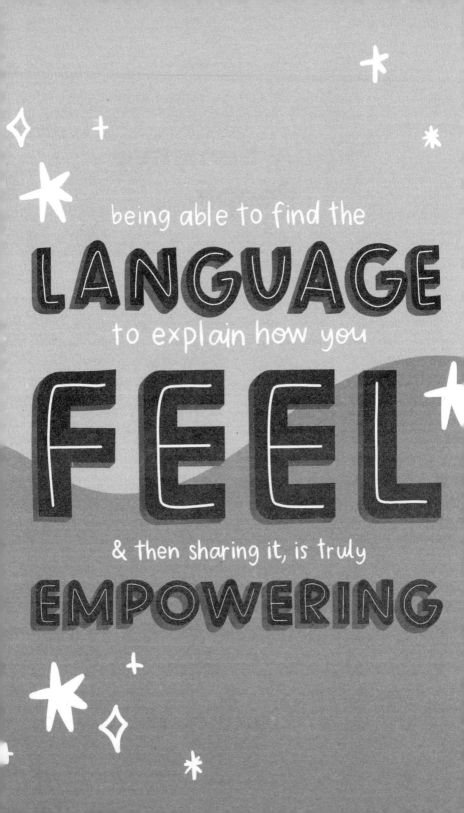

being able to find the

LANGUAGE

to explain how you

FEEL

& then sharing it, is truly

EMPOWERING

When I first discovered the concept of highly sensitive people, it felt like a real eureka moment. I wanted to call everyone immediately – my boyfriend, my mum, my cousin, my friends, my boss – and say: 'Look! This is me! Do you *see* now?'

Suddenly, everything made sense. I finally had an explanation for why I'd spent my whole life feeling . . . different. And, very quickly, I came to see it as a strength – in fact, I love being highly sensitive and I think I'd be a robot without it.

It was Dr Elaine Aron who first coined and pioneered the term, back in the 1990s, and while there has been a decent amount of research around it since, there's still not an awful lot of us clinical psychologists who know about it. Because of this, much of the treatment and intervention for things like anxiety and depression doesn't take into account the HSP trait, and I think that's a real shame because it can have a huge impact on your everyday life from the moment you open your eyes. I'd be doing many of you an injustice if I didn't give you the opportunity to learn a bit more about it.

Why *is* there such a lack of knowledge about it? Well, some clinical psychologists would say they're concerned about giving people another 'label'. Um, no, honey. My HSP label is one I wear with pride! Being able to experience people's emotions and reflect on that is perfect for my job – I literally work the highly sensitive magic and truly engage!

It's not the same sort of label as 'depression' or 'PTSD'. This is a personality trait and, by acknowledging it, all we're doing is saying: 'Welcome to the gang!'

Because, once we get it working properly, HSPs can soar.

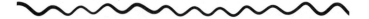

Are you a highly sensitive person?

Have a look at the twenty-seven statements below. If fourteen or more of them apply to you, then the chances are you're highly sensitive.

→ I am easily overwhelmed by strong sensory input.
→ I seem to be aware of subtleties in my environment.
→ Other people's moods affect me.
→ I tend to be very sensitive to pain.
→ I find myself needing to withdraw during busy days, into bed or a darkened room or any place where I can have some privacy and relief from stimulation.
→ I am particularly sensitive to the effects of caffeine.
→ I am easily overwhelmed by things like bright lights, strong smells, coarse fabrics or sirens close by.

→ I have a rich, complex inner life.

→ I am made uncomfortable by loud noises.

→ I am deeply moved by the arts or music.

→ My nervous system sometimes feels so frazzled that I just have to go off by myself.

→ I am conscientious.

→ I startle easily.

→ I get rattled when I have a lot to do in a short amount of time.

→ When people are uncomfortable in a physical environment, I tend to know what needs to be done to make it more comfortable (like changing the lighting or the seating).

→ I am annoyed when people try to get me to do too many things at once.

→ I try hard to avoid making mistakes or forgetting things.

→ I make a point of avoiding violent movies and TV shows.

→ I become unpleasantly aroused when a lot is going on around me.

→ Being very hungry creates a strong reaction in me, disrupting my concentration or mood.

→ Changes in my life shake me up.

→ I notice and enjoy delicate or fine scents, tastes, sounds, works of art.

→ I find it unpleasant to have a lot going on at once.

→ I make it a high priority to arrange my life to avoid upsetting or overwhelming situations.

→ I am bothered by intense stimuli, like loud noises or chaotic scenes.

→ When I must compete or be observed while performing a task, I become so nervous or shaky that I do much worse than I would otherwise.

→ When I was a child, my parents or teachers seemed to see me as sensitive or shy.

If you're ticking a lot of those boxes, don't worry! I know things have been hard for you, but guess what? We've just found your superpower.

What does it all mean?

According to the research done so far, as many as 15–20 per cent of us have the HSP trait. Yep, there are a lot of us out there! The technical term for it is Sensory Processing Sensitivity, and studies show the nervous system is different, not only making HSPs more susceptible to disorders if they've experienced trauma, but also meaning they process everything on a deeper level.

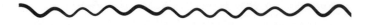

according to research done so far, ★ as many as 15-20% of us ✝ ★ ✝ ★ have the HSP trait ★ ✝

So, what people say to them, what they hear on the news, what they read – that can all feel like really heavy stuff. In crowds or spaces where there are lots of people talking at and around them, they may easily become overwhelmed and overstimulated by the sights, sounds, chatter, movement, smells and lights.

It might not make the HSP change anything they're doing, but they'll notice it, a hundred per cent.

They might, however, feel the need to slip out for a bit to re-energize, not because they don't like people or feel anxious, but because it's a lot to have to process.

As a child, I often felt anxious and afraid, like I was always ready for something to happen. I just felt everything so intensely – I still do. You know when people say kids are older than their years? I used to get that a lot, because I was always very conscious of other people's emotions around me. If I ever saw someone upset, even about the littlest thing, it would hurt me to the core. People would be like: 'Michaela, why do these things bother you?' And I wouldn't really have an answer beyond: 'I don't know, it just does! Why *doesn't* it bother you?'

Now I know it's the HSP thing and that I've spent a lifetime processing stuff on a different level and noticing things other people do not. Don't get me wrong, I was a happy child, but whenever I was around people it was a *lot*. Being highly sensitive is exhausting.

I remember when I was about nine, I went to Spain on holiday with my family. There was hotel entertainment in the evening and they had a Velcro wall where the hotel

Highly Sensitive Personality

What people THINK it means:

emotionally fragile

always over-reacting

weak

can't take a joke

What it REALLY means:

loyal

attuned to the needs of others

intuitive

creative thinker

cares deeply

guests could volunteer to put on a special suit and take a run-up, then jump and try to stick to the wall. Everyone was having a good time and laughing hysterically as people tried and sometimes failed. I, on the other hand, thought the whole thing was just so mean and I got so upset I had to leave. I went up to the hotel room and couldn't stop thinking about the people who hadn't managed it and how they would be sad the next day because people had been laughing at them. I couldn't shake it. I vividly remember that now, more than twenty years later.

How it can affect day-to-day life

To get an idea of what it feels like to be an HSP, take everything the average person thinks about on a daily basis and then double it both in terms of intensity and the length of time it's on your mind for.

OK, you're about halfway there.

It's having extreme sensitivities to the subtleties. So, people's facial expressions or a slight dip in temperature (if I feel so much as a tiny draught, I'm like: 'Urgh! Winter is here!') or the smell of food that is close to its sell-by date. It's not necessarily stuff that's going to cause you an issue, it's things you notice anyway.

All that can feel tiring because your senses are constantly working overtime. But the biggest hurdle to overcome is making sure none of that sensory processing is processing in the wrong direction and being used to reinforce your negative core beliefs. More on that shortly.

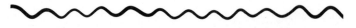

Signs your mind is overstimulated

→ You feel unable to take in any new information.
→ You can't tolerate loud noises, bright lights or other types of sensory stressors.
→ You feel tired even when you've had enough sleep.
→ Everyday chores like washing dishes feel overwhelming.
→ Your to-do list seems unbearable even when you'd usually be able to manage it.
→ You can't focus and feel irritable.

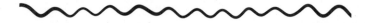

I think this would be a good point to acknowledge that there are some aspects of HSP that overlap with neurodevelopmental diagnoses such as Attention Deficit Hyperactivity Disorder (ADHD) and autism, and mental health disorders such as Post Traumatic Stress Disorder (PTSD). However, the devil is in the detail of the diagnostic criteria for each. For example, while the sensory sensitivity that is a big marker of autism is also key to HSP, in order to receive a diagnosis of Autism Spectrum Disorder (ASD) there are many other criteria involved, which HSP may or may not meet.

✦ ⸗CASE STUDy⸗ ✦

Lucy is at a big work event and has just entered the con-
ference hall, where everyone is enjoying drinks, canapés
and networking. There's talking, the lights are bright and
the temperature is warm. Too warm. All five of Lucy's
senses are picking up on and absorbing everything and
working overtime. She's perfectly able to connect with
people, hold conversations and keep people engaged but
it feels overwhelming.

The vibe in the room is overpowering. She senses the
need to get out.

Can you relate to Lucy's situation? I can! I used to hold my
breath when walking past people in a crowd – not because
they smelled bad but because I knew whatever I was going
to get a whiff of was going to feel too intense. I didn't
want to smell anything, not even if it was Chanel No 5.

In a scenario like this, it's totally fine for Lucy to readjust
her environment and 'tap out' for a while, that is, temporarily
remove herself. We know that, as an HSP, her nervous system is wired differently and so she shouldn't have to put
herself in the same situations as everyone else. When you're
highly sensitive and you feel overwhelmed, tapping out is a
perfectly acceptable response, not least because if you remain
in that situation for too long, it could potentially turn into
anxiety.

Now, I should mention here that tapping out when you
actually *do* feel anxious is very different and isn't necessarily

when you're HIGHLY SENSITIVE & feel OVERWHELMED, tapping out is a perfectly acceptable response...

the best course of action. In these instances, facing your fears – otherwise known as exposure – is better. So it's important to notice and learn what overwhelm (as opposed to anxiety) looks and feels like for you in terms of your thought processes, emotions and body. If that's what you're experiencing, take yourself out of that situation. You don't need to be there.

People often don't feel like they deserve to prioritize themselves enough to be able to change things, but readjusting your environment is about establishing some boundaries around your energy and it can have a transformative effect on your whole mindset. I'm going to give you a couple of really good grounding techniques that will help you tap out, bring it back and reduce those feelings of overwhelm. These are especially handy for situations that you can't physically leave – like a noisy plane journey.

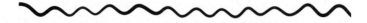

The 5–4–3–2–1 method

This will help to bring you back to the present moment. Stop whatever you're doing and name:

50

→ 5 things you can see
→ 4 things you can touch
→ 3 things you can hear
→ 2 things you can smell
→ 1 thing you can taste

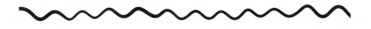

If you're feeling anxious, box breathing is a really useful technique to help relieve stress.

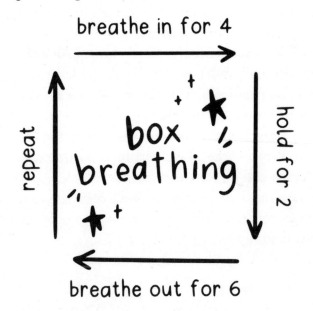

Being highly sensitive in the workplace

HSPs tend to be conscientious, meticulous about detail and hard workers, and all these attributes tend to go a long way when it comes to a career. There's also a strong aversion to disappointing people, and that can often result in getting good roles and doing very well in them.

At first glance, that might sound great. But it's not exactly, because the *motivation* behind all that is wrong and needs looking at. Being an overachiever because you don't want to disappoint people puts you at risk of eventually burning out.

'Oh, I've done a good job and you want to give me more work? Bring it on. Ooh, even more? OK . . . that's fine.'

I'm guessing that might be ringing a few bells.

The emotions HSPs take *in* are one thing, but the ones they actually experience themselves are ridiculously powerful, so they really don't want to feel the impact of saying no and will do pretty much anything to avoid it, even if that makes life harder for themselves in the long run.

'This is my thing. I do good work. And the alternative is to crumble to the floor, and then no one is going to respect me and I'll have to leave out of shame.'

Believe me, I've been there. We'll come on to this a lot more in Chapter 6, on people-pleasing, so hold on to your hats for that.

* =CASE STUDY= +

Farzana is approached by her boss about a report she's written and asked to add something to it that she's missed. She smiles, nods and says she'll get straight on it. But, inside, she's kicking herself: 'Argh, I missed it! How could

I have forgotten? I didn't do a good enough job. I'm use-less at this and now everyone is going to know it.'

Instead of quickly adding in the information her boss has very politely requested, Farzana is starting to over-think. The rabbit hole has opened up ready for her, and because she's interested in anything in line with her nega-tive core beliefs, in she jumps and down she goes.

Farzana isn't even thinking about how she can add a couple of lines into the report to make it better. She's thinking: 'What does this piece of (very neutral) feedback mean *now*? Are they going to tell anyone? What are they saying about me? What do they *think* about me?'

This is completely unproductive and energy-sapping. Learning how to take feedback is hard for HSPs but, sorry, guys, it's a necessary part of life. Whether it's feed-back or a nerve-wracking work meeting or anything else, always keep in mind the end game. What do you want to happen here? What do you want the outcome to be?

So Farzana's short-term goal for the outcome of this feedback should be to take it on board, improve the report and move on to whatever's next. She needs to focus on that and whether the thought process she's having right now is going to take her towards it or away from it. That's the choice.

In that moment, she could do a quick assessment.

I could *give my attention to my negative thoughts, and I* could *act in this way, but let me think about the end game and see how the line of thinking I'm going down helps me to get there.*

Now, it might be that it doesn't help because it's nothing to do with the situation at hand. Or it might be that it does have something to do with it but it makes her feel awful and triggers a really uncomfortable emotion that she hasn't yet learned to manage without a struggle. And feeling awful is going to make it so much harder for Farzana, or anyone in a similar position, to get to that end game.

So, notice when you're going down the rabbit hole, recognize you're at the choice point and make a decision. Any thought process that takes you *towards* where you want to be, go with that. It must be about what *you* think is valuable and whatever is in line with your personal values.

If that gets you to your end game? Cool, do your thing.

I'm not saying it won't be tricky. When the negative thoughts start up some lucky so-and-sos are able to say: '*Stop!*' in their head, and that works for them, but don't worry if it doesn't for you. I know only too well that telling yourself to stop thinking about something often makes you think about it even more. You know 'Don't think about the pink elephant!' means you instantly see a pink elephant bouncing about the living room.

It's less about trying to stop yourself thinking about that thing and more about finding something else to redirect your focus to and using as many of your senses as you can to zoom in on that. Some people keep an elastic band on their wrist and flick it when they notice they're overthinking, and that helps bring the focus back while they find something else to absorb their attention into.

That's where mindfulness comes in. It doesn't have to be anything spectacular, it could literally just be the pen you're holding. What does it smell like, feel like? What colour is it? The unhelpful thought might still be there at the back of your mind, and that's OK. Just let it be. Your conscious attention has been redirected to something else and – bingo! – you're moving towards your end game.

Honesty is the best policy

Creating an environment where you have the language to explain how you're feeling, especially with your bosses and colleagues, that is the holy grail. If you felt able to say to them, 'I really want to do a good job on this, but at the moment I'm feeling a bit overwhelmed so can I gather my thoughts and come back to it in a bit?', then how cool would that be?

Sending an honest email to your boss in this instance can be really helpful. Having said that, I had an HSP client who wrote this brilliant email, laying it all out to her boss about how she was feeling. But when the boss phoned her about it, she didn't pick up! So then she was suffering with the double stress of, first, how her boss was going to respond to the email and, second, the fact that she hadn't answered the call.

There's a lot of shame attached to being a high-achieving HSP because you have this very 'together' exterior and you want to maintain that. People don't know you're struggling, and that's a Good Thing, as far as you're concerned. But life is *so* much easier when people know. Shame lives in the dark and, when you start talking, you'll be surprised when nobody shuns you. If people care enough (and most of them do), they will adapt the way they operate around you.

You could give them prompts such as: 'I'd like a bit more time when we're working on this because I feel pressured with tight deadlines or being observed.' Or: 'If there's any way you could tell me in advance about projects that are coming up so I can start getting my mind into gear, that would be really helpful for me.'

Even something like: 'It might seem like I'm about to collapse in a crying heap on the floor when you give me feedback, but don't stop! I'm hearing it, I just process it a bit differently to what you might expect' is better than stewing on it, becoming defensive and having the person giving that feedback going away feeling that they can't have an open conversation with you.

Being able to find the language to explain how you feel, then sharing it, is truly empowering.

How being highly sensitive can affect relationships

We're all capable of being a bit over-analytical when we've got a new hottie in our lives. Scrutinizing texts is one thing. The HSP, on the other hand, will be noticing everything from a twitch in the eyebrows to someone stepping forward a bit differently and trying to work out what it could all possibly mean. All that stuff can make things very complicated internally.

Now, this doesn't mean it's an issue. It's not nice when you don't feel good inside, but what's important is making sure your actions aren't in line with anything unhelpful going on in your head. So, you might be analysing and scanning for signs about whether they like you or not, or if things have changed since the last time you saw them. And seriously? That's a lot of energy, and you should probably stop doing it. But it's not going to be a problem in the relationship unless you're using your new 'information' to reinforce your negative core beliefs.

On top of this, feedback can cause issues in relationships. We've already discussed that when people are giving an HSP feedback that's not wholly positive – even if it's just neutral – they're going to take it in and potentially process it as criticism. Not because of anything to do with the HSP's ego but because the empathy side of being highly sensitive hates to disappoint and wants to make the people around them happy. And if the HSP then starts reacting in an unhelpful way based on how they feel because of that feedback (hello, sulky face silent treatment) . . . well, that's when friction can occur in a relationship.

If feedback always makes someone upset, then the person giving it might end up being reluctant to speak, meaning they're then stuck with concerns they can't share. Not healthy.

We're going deep

A common characteristic found in HSPs is deep processing. We are able to process information in a complex way, understanding the meaning or intention behind words and ideas, rather than taking them at face value. HSPs like to analyse problems from multiple angles and will probably pursue various solutions to form a full picture of what is in front of them.

This deep processing usually takes time and this means that HSPs can take longer to arrive at a decision, especially if there is a lot of information. This doesn't always lead to overthinking, but the state of extended focus can contribute to difficulties in thinking clearly.

If you're an HSP, in addition to processing information deeply, you will often seek to maximize the amount of information you take in at any given time. This might be done as a way to figure out how best react to or understand the world around you, but it can also quickly lead to information overwhelm. With social media and access to virtually anything on the internet, many HSPs get confused or overwhelmed by the multitude of information out there.

As HSPs, it may seem that maximizing information intake is helping us make an informed decision, but it often leads us to avoid decision-making completely due to overthinking every single aspect. Decision fatigue is real, people! HSPs want to make the best decision, find the best option and make sure everyone is happy, and this can be a lot of pressure, leading to an inability to take action.

There may come a point where a decision simply needs to be made in order to move forward. It can be very difficult to feel like you are settling for anything less than the best, but keep in mind that you are naturally skilled at analysing and coming to conclusions, so trust your gut and don't let your anxiety make you question yourself more than necessary.

STRENGTHS
OF HSP

- Able to make deep connections with others
- Experiencing positive emotions on another level
- High attention to detail
- Fabulous creativity and deep rich thought
- Deep intuition and instinct
- Highly perceptive to other people's emotions
- Can experience really strong positive emotions from the arts, and nature
- Thrives in quiet calm environments
- Enjoys being able to find quiet after feeling frequently emotionally exhausted

HSPs and empathy

HSPs are natural empaths and are highly aware of the feelings of others around them. When making decisions, we keep the wants and needs of others in mind and tend to prioritize them over our own. We also usually fear disappointing others, for example cancelling plans with a friend even though we're not feeling well and need to rest.

While empathy can be a strength in many situations, it can lead HSPs down a spiral of overthinking and worry that is usually entirely unnecessary. It is important for HSPs to find a balance between understanding the needs of others while prioritizing themselves and their well-being. If you find yourself prioritizing other people's feelings or opinions in your decision-making process, take a second to reconnect with your mind and body. Consider each of the options and see how you react. Ask yourself if you truly want to attend that party this evening. If you feel energized, go and have fun! If your body feels tired, it's telling you to rest, and your friends will understand.

The best bits about being an HSP

I promise you, there is *so* much to love about being highly sensitive, and it's not something you should ever apologize for. The world needs people with your amazing sensitivity!

* the world NEEDS more people *.
with your AMAZING sensitivity!

I like to think of HSPs existing because we're needed to stop the less sensitive people running off into danger. That's our place in terms of evolution, according to Elaine Aron. Sure, you might be seen as a Cautious Cathy, but a bit of caution is necessary in certain situations. We need people to have the foresight to say: 'Er, hang on, let's just think about this. Can we slow down a bit, analyse and plan?'

You care about the things you do; you naturally pay attention to detail and you genuinely want to do a good job. Being an HSP also means you are great at problem-solving, you are creative and have an ability to see things from different angles. In a team environment, it's useful to notice any changes and look for gaps and put a creative spin on them. Being able to read the room can put you one step ahead of everyone else, and that is super-useful.

You can tell when people are off. You can even tell when animals are off! My Russian Blue cats Luna and Winter? I can read them like a book.

But it's empathy that is the absolute best part of being highly sensitive – the connection you can have with people and how comfortable you can make them feel. You're the person people want to come to for emotional support. And for me personally, this is where I feel that I shine.

How to reclaim your energy as an HSP

Constantly thinking, feeling and processing deeply is exhausting, so you have to make a conscious effort to notice which environments deplete your energy. Then you can set some flexible rules about how you manage or avoid these environments. After all, you can't keep jumping into the frying pan and expecting not to get burnt, so let's switch things up a bit.

You could start with setting a boundary around how long you stay at family gatherings without a break or by asking your boss to identify a quiet space for you to get away from a noisy co-worker. If you hate noisy, boisterous crowds, then you might plan to stay away from the next party. If you usually process and overthink the emotions, feelings and facial expression of others, you might want to spend less time with unkind or passive-aggressive people who give you more negative stimuli to process and more things to over-think about when you get home. (Why did she raise her eyebrow when she said that? What did she really mean when she told me this? Does she hate me?)

Don't jam-pack your diary to the point where you have no breathing time to process your experiences through-out the week. You will benefit from this time to mull over, problem-solve, sit with and enjoy the past week's shenanigans.

And please, please, please, tidy something – go full-on Marie Kondo in your spaces if you can, because clutter and mess are not your friends. But you already knew that.

What to do now?

Honestly? Accept it and have compassion for yourself. This is who you are! It is what you are. We are not seeking to change this part of ourselves and, in fact, you'd be doing yourself and the people around you a disservice if you did.

What we *do* have to think about changing is the narrative. Recognize this as a positive thing and speak to other people in terms of it being just that. Sure, there are certain struggles, but we're not going to lead with the struggle. However, in order to be more productive, we need to get really good at discerning what needs our attention and what doesn't, and then letting go of those unhelpful thoughts that lead us nowhere.

That's easier said than done, but practising and perfecting the mindfulness skill is literally the antidote to intrusive thoughts. It's a bit like going to the gym – getting fit isn't just going to happen on its own, you have to keep going, but once you've got into that habit and learned that skill, it's invaluable. Training your brain in this way will allow you to decide at any point what you need to focus your attention on.

Distracted? That's OK, because we can bring it back.

This is really important for HSPs, because of the sheer amount of processing going on inside us. When it comes to taking something and running with it for a long time and lifting it to a level where it really doesn't need to be, we are world-beaters. And that can be quite time-consuming as well.

As a human being, you are going to experience uncomfortable emotions and sensations, and that's OK too. It's about learning to accept them and not trying to do things for the rest of your life to try and avoid them. The Acceptance and Commitment Therapy (ACT) model tells us that life is hard and, while there will be great moments, we should not always be striving for happiness, because that's what keeps us suffering.

The difficult emotions are painful – no one is saying they're not – but consistently trying to avoid them is turning that pain into suffering. The end goal is to have psychological flexibility, and this is going to be key throughout this book. That means experiencing any thought or feeling and still being able to move in the direction of your values and what's important to you.

Don't allow those unhelpful thoughts and uncomfortable emotions to throw you off track. Emotions are not going to kill you – they're designed to keep you alive. I'm going to get you to a point where you can sit with them, even lean into them a bit, and still do what you need to do.

CHAPTER THREE

Anxiety

'The body keeps the score.'

– Bessel van der Kolk

note to self:

YOU DON'T HAVE TO LIVE LIKE THIS!*

* there are things you can do to get anxiety under control and feel better able to deal with triggering situations.

OK, so let's start this off with the facts: you are so not alone in this. Everyone has anxiety, and anyone who says they don't is either lying or not aware of what anxiety is! Regardless of age, sex, whether you're introvert or extrovert, rich or poor, you can't escape experiencing some form of anxiety at some point in your life.

What is anxiety?

When it comes to mental health conditions, we clinicians tend to do a lot of categorizing. Identifying and grouping common concerns and symptoms helps us to plan treatment, and there are a few mental health disorders that fall under the broad umbrella of anxiety disorders. The most prevalent of these are generalized anxiety disorder and social anxiety.

Generalized anxiety disorder shows up as super-excessive worrying (we'll address this in Chapter 4, on overthinking), whereas social anxiety shows up as an intense fear of being judged by your peers and those around you.

Other anxiety disorders include health anxiety, phobias and body dysmorphic disorder. Oh, and obsessive compulsive disorder, panic disorder and Post Traumatic Stress Disorder . . . Trust me when I say the list could go on.

Clinicians don't go around making up disorders and the criteria for them. We use our clinical judgement and a manual (thank God for manuals!) called the Diagnostic and Statistical Manual of Mental Disorders (DSM) and/or the International Classification of Diseases (ICD), where you'll find every mental health disorder known to man mentioned, if you feel inclined to look them up!

Just like any physical health condition, the symptoms of anxiety disorders will vary from person to person. You might experience anxiety attacks that come on without warning, while Jessica gets panicky at the mere thought of talking to people at a party. Seemingly confident Debbie may struggle with a disabling fear of driving or uncontrollable thoughts, while your boss might live in a constant state of tension, worrying about anything and everything.

What all these responses have in common is an intense fear or worry that very probably doesn't match up to the actual situation. Struggling with anxiety or having a diagnosis of an anxiety disorder can prevent you from living the life you want, but it's entirely possible to turn it around. Once you understand the nature of your anxiety, there are steps that you can take to reduce the symptoms and get back in control. We're going to cover these in this chapter.

struggling with anxiety or having a
diagnosis of an anxiety disorder *
* can <u>prevent</u> you from living the *
life you want, but it's entirely
* <u>possible</u> to turn it around.
*

High-functioning anxiety (HFA)

There's one extremely common anxiety problem that hasn't been classified as a disorder, and that's high-functioning anxiety.

Women with HFA (hey, me!) know how to keep busy, they thrive on achieving the highest level of perfection in their work and life and they have an extreme need for control in their lives. These people are driven by details, mostly in an attempt to calm the racing thoughts and fears that invade their mind. Those around them often don't know they're struggling with any of this, of course, because it's all hidden beneath a beautiful mask of achievement. Except it's anxiety that's driving the achievement.

Sustainable? Nope. But that's what this book is for.

Anxiety and evolution

Remember when I said everyone has anxiety? Well, that's not completely true, there *is* a group of people that doesn't have anxiety – dead people. Dead people don't have anxiety. Too harsh? OK, maybe, but I never did master the sugarcoating thing.

Now, if you're reading this book, then you, my friend, are very much alive. So well done! And believe it or not, your anxiety is one of the main reasons why this is the case . . . allow me to explain.

Anxiety feels awful – your heart beats faster, you sweat, you're plagued with butterflies, an upset stomach and, during a full-blown anxiety attack, you're certain that you're either about to have a heart attack, 'go crazy' or die. But you never *actually* die, or have a heart attack or 'go crazy', do you? So what's really going on? Well, your threat response has been activated and your body is basically doing its job in fighting the threat and protecting you, albeit too eagerly.

Now let's take it back – wayyyy back.

Millions of years ago (think Stone Age years ago) our brains and bodies evolved and developed special automatic mechanisms to keep us alive. You might think life is hard now, but the dangers back then? Sheesh!

In order to have a chance at surviving in the prehistoric environment, humans had to be super-vigilant for threats and even better at avoiding any danger coming their way. Our default setting was safety first.

Fast-forward to today, and have things changed? Well, no. Our automatic survival mechanism is still fully present (we call it the threat response) and our brains are still alerting us to things that might hurt us. Except now it's not sabre-toothed tigers that are the threat, it's presentations at work, a cough lasting a little too long, an argument with a friend or ordering a Subway sandwich (again, no judgement; it is what it is).

So, our brain has been alerted to a potential threat – now what?

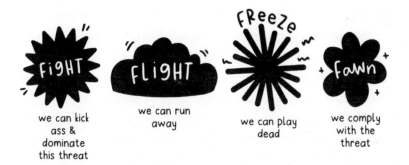

we can kick ass & dominate this threat

we can run away

we can play dead

we comply with the threat

Once we've detected a threat, we have to do something about it.

These reactions don't just happen. Instead, something really interesting occurs before we take any action at all. I can't remember if I was ever taught this in biology (I can't remember most of what I was taught in biology, tbh) but, nonetheless, I'm about to get real geeky here and give you a super-quick science lesson. So bear with me.

There are several key players in our brain that take complete control in moments of potential threat and then work together to keep us safe and out of harm's way. The first is the amygdala, a part of the brain that helps process emotion. When we're confronted with a potential threat, our eyes and ears send a signal to the amygdala. If it interprets the images and sounds as dangerous, it sends a message to our second key player, the hypothalamus, saying something along the lines of: 'Quick! Danger!'

Think of the hypothalamus as the Big Boss – it's essentially the command centre that communicates with the rest of our body through the third key player, the autonomic nervous system (ANS). The ANS controls the next two key players: the sympathetic nervous system (SNS) and the parasympathetic nervous system (PNS). The SNS kicks off some major, but temporary, physical changes that enable us to run, fight or play dead.

These changes are literally head to toe. You might not even notice all of them, but they are happening. This very efficient team is called the limbic system. Are you still awake? Good! There's more . . .

These changes triggered by the limbic system happen rapidly – our brains and bodies are wired together so well that before the brain's visual centres have a chance to cotton on to what's happening, the amygdala and hypothalamus are already working tirelessly to keep us safe. In a life-or-death situation, we don't have the time to go back and forward processing information – that's where our survival mechanism kicks in so we can respond before we've even thought about what we're doing.

A lot of the anxiety we feel is because there *should* be a threat to life – and, if there was, we'd be running away from it or fighting it, right? But instead, you're usually just sitting there with it, so one of the things I tell people to do is to move their body. Jump up and down. Do ten star jumps. Pretend you're Beyoncé playing 'Single Ladies' live

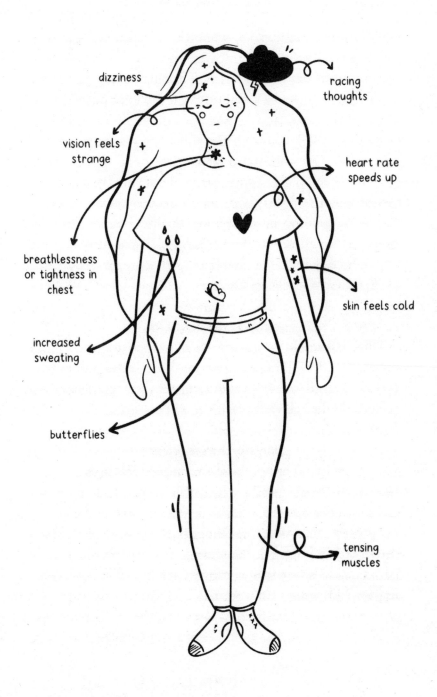

at Wembley Stadium – whatever it takes to get you moving.

Your body has this energy but, because whatever's going on is not 'technically' a real threat, it can't get rid of it.

What's going on?

Anxiety can feel ten times worse when you don't know what's happening in your body or understand why. I'm going to break down the physical changes most people experience, which feel awful but, in a life-or-death situation, are extremely functional.

Heart rate speeds up

All the tissues in our body need oxygen to work more effectively; this increase in your heart rate pumps the blood around your body a little faster so it can deliver the oxygen to the relevant places more promptly.

Skin starts to feel cold;
tingling or numbness in fingers and toes

Our SNS is so sophisticated it will immediately reorganize blood flow to the areas that need it most and divert it away from areas like your fingers (your SNS really isn't interested in your gel manicure), toes or your skin, none of which, let's face it, are going to help you if a car is coming towards you at full speed.

Breathlessness and chest pain and/or tightness

Breathing speeds up and gets deeper in order to take in enough oxygen to enable us to carry out the action we need to take. There's no 'comfortable' way for our bodies to do this, so it leaves us breathless or with tightness or pain in the chest, and for some, it can feel as if we're legit choking.

Dizziness

A by-product of that extra breathing is the blood supply to the head decreasing. Don't be alarmed – just like all the other things on the list, this isn't dangerous, but it does feel very unpleasant. Getting hot flushes and feeling a bit detached from reality at these times isn't uncommon either, for the same reasons. Wild, right?

Increase in sweating

The increase in sweat cools the body so it doesn't start overheating and pack up. Not only that, imagine you are really in a fight or need to escape a predator – if you're all sweaty and slippery, it's going to be much harder for the predator to get hold of you. You can just glide on right out of there. Granted, if the threat that triggers your SNS is a meeting with your boss and you start sweating like crazy, then that's not so good. But if it's any consolation, it does mean that your automatic survival mechanism is working well so, you know, every cloud!

Vision gets weird

When your SNS is triggered, your pupils dilate to let in more light. In this scenario you may start feeling that the lights are too bright, or your vision gets blurry, or you might even see spots. This is all going on because your vision is trying to become more acute so that you can pay more attention to the threat.

Racing thoughts

Your thinking needs to speed up so you can make quicker decisions to avoid the approaching threat. You can't think of anything but the danger, and for good reason – you need to fight that scary thing or get out of there, or else, as far as your ANS is concerned, you will surely die!

Butterflies and/or needing the toilet urgently

This is the worst one for me personally. If you're in the midst of danger, you really don't need to waste energy on your digestive system, so your ANS tells it to slow down – energy can be diverted to systems in your body that are more helpful in escaping the imminent threat. I literally stopped eating brown toast for brekkie as I kept getting bubble guts and thought I was allergic, but later I realized I was just anxious at work.

Tensing up

There's no time for relaxation or sleep when you're in danger. Your body needs to stay ready for action so your muscles start preparing for the showdown and tense up.

It's not uncommon to feel aches and pains, trembling and shaking, especially if you're standing still.

As you can see, the process involved in our wonderfully evolved automatic survival mechanism – the threat response – is major. Everything works together divinely, but all the physical changes in your body can leave you feeling exhausted and, if you don't understand what's happening, even more scared than when you noticed the original threat. The main thing to remember here – and the most reassuring – is that you won't die; your body is just doing what it needs to do to keep you safe. I mean, we would be a very inefficient species if the thing that was designed to keep us alive actually killed us!

If you were in a life-or-death situation, you probably wouldn't notice many of these bodily changes because you'd already be running or fighting or playing dead. But those of us who get anxiety from posting social media pictures or speaking on the phone feel this while sitting on our butts or walking down the street. We're left with all this energy and all these hyped-up body functions but no actual threat to use them on.

Very uncomfortable, to say the least.

Getting back to baseline

So your flight response has been triggered and you've managed to escape that scary thing. Now what? Now, it's key player number three's time to shine.

This one is known as the parasympathetic nervous system, and it's just as important as the sympathetic nervous system, but for different reasons. The PNS is the system that's going to get you out of survival mode and back to your relaxed state. Once the coast is clear and you're out of harm's way, your ANS instructs your PNS to essentially counteract everything the SNS is doing.

No more racing heart rate and shallow breathing, your temperature begins to lower and your muscles start to relax. Think of the SNS as an accelerator pedal in a car; it triggers the 'threat response' to give you that burst of energy to deal with the perceived danger in front of you. If the SNS is the accelerator, the PNS is the brake that triggers the 'rest and digest response' that helps bring you back down again.

You're probably thinking, 'OK, so that makes sense in theory, but why do I still feel anxious even when I can see that the threat is gone?'

Well, it doesn't make sense to relax immediately, as we can't be *sure* the threat is gone. In caveman days, even if that sabre-toothed tiger backed off, it might come back again, so we would have needed to stay prepared for a little longer, just in case. That's why our anxiety tapers off only gradually, giving us time to make sure the coast is clear before we fully relax.

The downside is that we have to experience the physical changes instructed by our survival mechanism for a little longer. But now you can understand why, even when the threat is gone, you might still feel a little revved up.

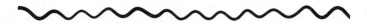

Thoughts = feelings = behaviour

Thoughts: 'If I go out, something bad might happen, I might embarrass myself. What if I see someone I know? What if my train gets delayed? I wouldn't be able to cope.'
Feelings: Anxiety.
Behaviour: Avoid going out, therefore not facing your fear or allowing yourself the opportunity to disprove your initial thought.

And then . . . the cycle starts back up the next time you might need to go out.
Waaahhhhhh!
So where are our exit points out of this torturous cycle??

Thoughts: Challenge them and/or accept them as just thoughts.
Behaviour: Do the opposite of what the anxious thoughts are telling you to do – go out in spite of those feelings. The quickest change comes from adjusting the behaviour, but it's also the hardest.

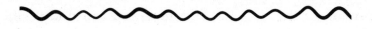

✳ ⹂CASE STUDY⹂ ✦

Sophie is due to give a presentation at work in front of the CEO of the company. A little bit of anxiety is fine, but she is off the scale with the whole: 'I can't do this, I'm going to mess up, everyone is watching me, I'm not going to be able to live this down, I'm going to lose my job and end up homeless.'

Yep, those thoughts sure can spiral.

She has a belly ache and is sweating. Sophie decides to phone in sick on the morning of the presentation.

Sophie could have those anxious thoughts and feelings and still do what she needed to do, but her behaviour is to opt out. The avoidance reduces the anxiety, but in avoiding the situation Sophie reinforces the initial negative thought that she can't do this.

The only way she can get rid of that negative thought is by having evidence against it, and she's not going to get that if she's doing the same avoidance thing over and over – in fact, all she's doing is creating even more unhelpful 'Why am I like this?' thoughts.

I know people at school used to say: 'Urgh, Michaela thinks she's better than everyone else. She doesn't like us, and we don't like her.'

But the truth was, I never knew what to say. I would go mute in a group and, because I was anxious, I wasn't smiling or engaged, and I guess it made me look aloof.

That was all part of my unhelpful cycle.

Thoughts: 'I don't think I have anything to say and people are going to judge me.'
Feeling: Anxiety.
Behaviour: Don't say anything at all.

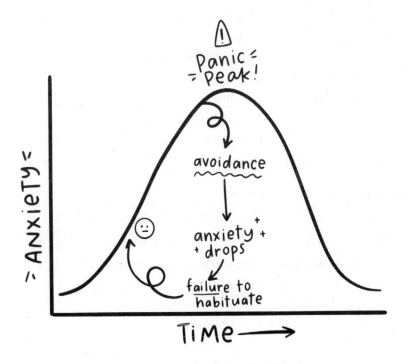

It created a situation which maintained the idea that people didn't like me, and it's so exhausting being trapped like that. Avoidance adds fuel to the fire and is one of the biggest structures in maintaining anxiety.

If Sophie had gone and done the presentation, her anxiety would have slowly gone down because adrenaline doesn't last that long in our body unless something else comes in and sets it off again. Doing that once won't suddenly make her fearless. Of course not. But it does mean that the next time, instead of the anxiety getting to a ten before going down, it might only reach an eight. And then she'll do it again and again until it's not something she's anxious about any more.

We heavily underestimate our ability to handle difficult situations, even though we do it time and time again. Go back and think about all the chaos and mayhem you've managed to deal with in your life – I bet you've forgotten most of it. You think you can't deal with it, but your history tells you that you can.

we **heavily** underestimate our ability to handle difficult situations even though we do it time and time again

The faulty car alarm

Now we know what's happening in our bodies when we feel anxious, hopefully that's one less thing to be anxious about. But what if our anxiety is getting in the way of living our everyday life, spending time with people we love or achieving things we know we're capable of? Why would the thing that's meant to keep us alive be making us so miserable?

I often liken our threat response to a car alarm. The car alarm has a job, and that's to deter people from stealing your car. In order to do this, it sits there quietly and, when it detects a potential robbery, it makes a loud noise to warn off the thieves.

That's like our threat response: it's always there, vigilant, waiting, not causing any trouble, just ready to do its job.

However, sometimes the car alarm develops a fault which means that even when someone lightly brushes past the car with no intention of stealing it, it starts sounding. We've all heard that car alarm going off at 3 a.m. for no apparent reason. For some of us, our threat response is like that faulty car alarm. We need it, but we only want it to work when there's a real threat. Our faulty car alarm (aka our sensitive threat response) has trouble identifying a real threat and a fake threat, so it ends up continuously ringing.

Living with anxiety happily

You don't have to live like this – there are things you can do to get anxiety under control and feel better able to deal with triggering situations.

Think of anxiety as your new BFF. Sometimes she'll show up unannounced. Sometimes she'll ask for your attention right before you're about to do something important. Sometimes you'll thank her and sometimes you'll never want to see her again. Deep down, you know you can't get through life without her, so here's how to make the journey better.

Over many years of working on the frontline in the NHS, and then through the last few years working with private clients, I have developed a combined system that I think is the most effective way to help the people I work with. I fuse together Cognitive Behavioural Therapy (CBT) and Acceptance and Commitment Therapy (ACT), which are two different models. CBT challenges the thoughts and ACT uses mindfulness to allow the thoughts to pass.

The first thing to do is to identify if this is a real threat or a fake threat (usually, it will be fake); then, use techniques to unhook yourself from those unhelpful thoughts. A car coming towards you at full speed? Real, obviously. Sending a risky message to the guy you met on Bumble? Fake. But if you decide it's a *real* threat, then you get all the bubble-guts stuff that comes with that.

We can't control the thoughts that come into our mind, but we can control which ones get our attention. I know it sounds quite hard to do at first, but the more you do it, the better you'll become at it.

we CAN'T control the thoughts
✦ that come into our minds, ✦
✦ but we CAN control which ✦
✦ ones get our attention! ✱

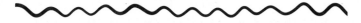

How to defuse your unhelpful thoughts

These techniques might sound *ridiculous*, but they help take the sting out of the thought – it stops being a 'fact' and becomes mere words. Singing it to the tune of 'Happy Birthday' is kinda funny, a little bit awkward, and it removes the intensity because you're basically just taking the p*ss out of it.

This is where mindfulness comes in as well – using judgement and just letting the thoughts pass.

→ Sing the thought to the tune of 'Happy Birthday'.
→ Picture the thought on a computer screen and blow it up, flip it around, zoom in and zoom out.
→ Picture the thoughts like leaves on a stream and just let them flow past you.
→ Put the thoughts on a cloud in the sky and let them float away.

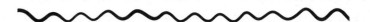

Yes, the thoughts are there and they can feel powerful, but we need to make sure that, in spite of how real they feel, we are putting our attention towards the things which take us in the direction of a meaningful life. The thoughts tempting you away from that are the ones you need to unhook yourself from.

You *should* be doing that presentation because it's in line with your professional goals. And if you know that, then the behaviour change also needs to happen. The worst thing we can do is avoid the presentation altogether. Or it could be bringing someone else in to help you do the presentation – sorry, but that's still avoiding.

Remember, no matter what your negative thoughts are telling you, choose goals that are in line with what you truly want and make sure the day-to-day behaviour leads up to that. Take the anxiety along with you if you need to, but don't avoid!

Quick win – in an anxious moment take a few slow deep breaths, remind yourself that you are safe, then ask yourself: 'If I was feeling super-confident right now how would I behave?' Close your eyes, imagine what that looks like, what that feels like . . . then do that!

Shout-out to the HSPs

Interestingly, the over arousal that comes with high sensitivity and the symptoms of anxiety are often confused. Dr Elaine Aron says that arousal may appear as blushing, trembling, heart pounding, hands shaking, foggy thinking, stomach churning, muscles tensing, and perspiring. This sounds a lot like the symptoms of anxiety I mentioned earlier, Right? So it's no wonder the two get mixed up.

According to Aron, once us highly sensitive people notice arousal, we want to know its source, and we often just assume we're anxious. We don't realize that our heart may be pounding from the sheer effort of processing extra stimulation. Or, other people assume we are afraid (given our obvious arousal), so we assume it too. Then, on deciding we must be afraid, the symptoms increase.

However, if fear isn't triggering these symptoms, then it isn't anxiety. As a rule, if you're feeling overwhelmed, it could be down to high sensitivity, and if you're feeling fear, then that is anxiety.

Let's take the networking event we talked about in Chapter 2, on highly sensitive people, but this time your thoughts are stuck on how people will judge you, especially because you're feeling flustered, and you worry they might notice, and what if you end up a Billy No Mates because no one wants to speak to you, and what if people see that you have no one to speak to, or you get into a conversation with someone who doesn't agree with your opinion and you're reminded of your awful ex-boss who used to gaslight you at every chance . . . well, now your body's threat response has been activated and you shut down. That is probably anxiety.

Particularly if you're a highly sensitive person, you really need to pay attention to these feelings and sensations and catch them early before they take over. And we do this by asking ourselves: am I feeling fear or is this overwhelm? If we decide that it is fear, the *next* question we need to ask is: real threat or fake threat?

Anxiety and trauma

Unfortunately, for many of us, our high levels of anxiety is the symptom of a trauma response. Post Traumatic Stress Disorder can develop after an experience of severe psychological distress following any terrible or life-threatening event.

In a super-basic nutshell, the memories of these events don't get processed in the same way as other memories, making them so much more easily triggered (think recurring nightmares of the event and flashbacks). It's a bit like having a messy cupboard. You open the doors, and it's just piles of clothes which you have to push back in to close the doors again. But as soon as something brushes past those doors, everything comes tumbling out because the cupboard is not in order.

That jumble is the trauma not being processed properly. If you took everything out of the cupboard, folded it up and put it back nicely, you could open and close it when you wanted to. Until the trauma is processed, we're going to carry on being triggered by it, whether that's on a big or a small level.

Our brains have specific triggers based on past traumatic events which aren't always obvious to us. If you experienced an accident as a child, such as almost drowning, it may develop into a seemingly irrational fear of water as an adult that you or the people around you don't understand, purely because of the unconscious manifestation of symptoms.

You only know that when you're around water you feel anxious – your past experience has programmed your brain's survival system to become overly sensitive to that particular 'threat'. This is because it's not about the memory, it's about how our bodies *perceive* that memory. Even long after the event has concluded, the memories of it are still so raw they can feel as if they are happening all over again, as if we're stuck in the past.

Remember, this survival system works rapidly and doesn't really allow time for logic, so if we're triggered as an adult, the rational thought that says we're safe now goes out of the window and in comes the flood of emotions and physical responses.

By becoming aware of your thought patterns, what triggers you to feel anxiety and where and how you feel it in your body, you learn to think, feel and act differently and start protecting yourself while healing from old, destructive wounds instead of reinforcing them.

Nearly every woman I speak to who is struggling with anxiety has some kind of memory which they can trace their anxiety back to. The spectrum of trauma can be anything from living through a car crash to having an invalidating environment growing up. For example, many women who were picked on at school struggle with social occasions – they feel anxious when they're out and they hate speaking in public, even if it's something they're actually really good at. It's not only the cognitive memories they can trace their anxiety back to but the physical memories too.

In fact, many psychologists agree that nervous system dysregulation can come from unresolved trauma within the body. Bestselling author Dr Bessel van der Kolk describes this well in the title of his book *The Body Keeps the Score*.

Everyone has a bundle of nerves in their brainstem that acts as a guard between their brain and their senses (sight, hearing, touch, and so on) and controls what information gets through to them and what doesn't.

It's called the Reticular Activating System (RAS), and we have this so we'll be motivated to behave in a certain way, ideally one that will keep us alive in the most automatic way possible. It filters through any information relevant to your survival and blocks the rest of the info to the point where you aren't even aware of it.

Dr Nicole LePera writes on her Instagram page: 'Our subconscious mind works to confirm our core beliefs in our environment. What we think about and believe to be true is filtered through . . . the RAS.'

It doesn't mean the evidence that you aren't really in danger isn't there, however, and, unfortunately for those with a trauma history, the information filtered through is based on their trauma rather than the reality of the current situation.

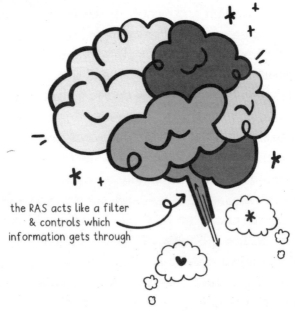

the RAS acts like a filter
& controls which
information gets through

This is why it's essential to challenge thoughts and let them go if they do not take us in the direction we want, rather than listening to them as fact.

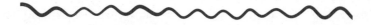

If you are experiencing anxiety as a result of a traumatic episode, seek professional help. Try to find a therapist who understands PTSD, abuse, developmental trauma or attachment trauma and can help you work through the original traumas, find coping mechanisms and get you on the path to recovery.

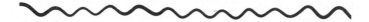

Get back to your body

Any trauma can impact our relationship with our bodies. Many of us cope with trauma by ignoring uncomfortable feelings, distracting ourselves from the present moment by doing other things, getting stuck in our heads and, essentially, dissociating. I know that word might sound a bit formal and scary, but stick with me – we'll get to what all this means as we move through the book together.

If you want true healing from the inside out, then as well as the more cognitive talking therapy, you have to add some focus back to your body. Even if that feels frightening.

This can be achieved through engaging in things like Eye Movement Desensitization and Reprocessing (EMDR), yin yoga, yoga therapy, breathwork, cold therapy, somatic therapy and body work – as well as super-quick day-to-day things like noticing your posture and making sure your body isn't tensed up (FYI, that indicates you're in threat mode), and unclenching your jaw. Or being more intentional about your breathing and, as a start, remembering to breathe!

I always used to hold my breath when I was anxious or trying to concentrate, and that would make me even more anxious. You can also practise noticing when you're holding your breath or using short and shallow anxious breaths so you can switch them to longer and slower inhales and exhales.

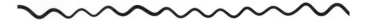

Try setting an alert on your phone for a particular time each day to do a body scan. Take a few slow, deep breaths from your belly, bringing your attention down to your feet, and see if you can notice any sensations, how you feel, where you're holding stress, and any thoughts or emotions that accompany it. Gently breathe through any tightness, pain or pressure. Then continue to scan your entire body in this way, gradually moving up from your feet until you reach the top of your head.

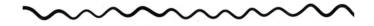

Getting back to your body isn't always easy, so expect some uncomfortable thoughts and feelings when doing these exercises, but the more you do them, the safer your body will begin to feel and the less heightened your emotional responses to certain triggers will be.

If your nervous system is dysregulated due to unresolved trauma in your body, then by shifting some focus to your body in this way you are helping to regulate your autonomic nervous system and increase its flexibility. This will reduce your overall anxiety and increase your ability to cope with what remains.

Speaking of your ANS, lots of research has been done into the role of the vagus nerve, vagal tone and its impact on mood. The vagus nerve is part of the ANS and a key nerve in the pathway of the parasympathetic nervous system (PNS). If you remember, the PNS is responsible for the body's relaxing response after a stressful situation.

Strong vagal tone is generally associated with a lower heart rate, better heart rate variability and being able to relax more quickly and easily after stress. Low vagal tone means the vagus nerve is not working as well as it could, which sometimes creates an overly heightened stress response. If that heightened stress response becomes chronic, we could experience things like anxiety, inflammation and gut issues.

Four things that have been shown to positively affect vagus tone are:

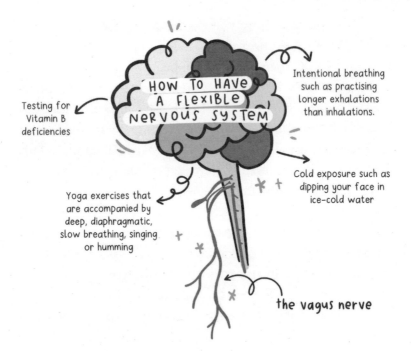

Mindfulness over matter

One of the most helpful forms of self-practice we can use to cope with anxiety is mindfulness. It's about learning to recognize, accept and feel our emotions early, before they take us over.

Journalling is another way to cope with anxiety. By writing down our emotions when we experience them, we are accepting them, enhancing our self-awareness and getting to the source of why we feel the way we do.

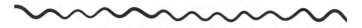

Tense and release

Tense and release is a progressive muscle relaxation exercise that helps bring awareness back to the body.

Go through every muscle you can imagine, starting with your eyebrows, your nose, your neck, your chin, your shoulders, all the way down to your big toes.

Hunch them up then drop them down, relaxing each part bit by bit.

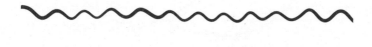

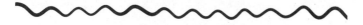

Belly breathing

When practising deep breathing, make sure to breathe slowly, from the belly, expanding your stomach, inhaling through your nose and exhaling through your mouth. The exhale triggers the relaxation response, so make sure to exhale for longer than you inhale. If it helps, breathe in for four seconds and breathe out for six.

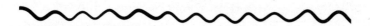

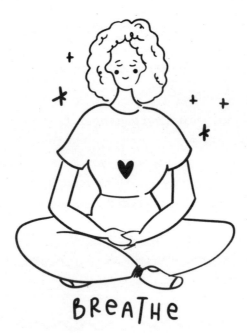

BREATHE

The plus side to anxiety – yes, there is one!

When it's managed properly, low-level anxiety can serve as a powerful tool and help you to put in extra effort towards something you care about. Research has reported that those who experience and manage anxiety can perform better creatively, in sports, in leadership roles, at job interviews and even while taking tests.

It's important to reframe our story – anxiety doesn't have to be seen as an inhibitor or as something negative. For example, people with social anxiety tend to be more understanding and empathetic because it's a heightened sense of caring. So, hey, it has its benefits! Don't let it stop you. Learn how to accept it, become aware of it early and see if you can use it to help you with your self-growth.

And the next time anxiety rolls up unannounced to hang out, acknowledge her, let her know how you feel about her and proceed in a way that is best to you.

After all, she's not in charge of your life, you are.

CHAPTER FOUR

Overthinking

'Overthinking doesn't solve problems,
it creates them.'

the scenarios you've created in your mind AREN'T real, BUT the time you've wasted thinking about them VERY much is!

Being an overthinker can feel like having an anxious parent in your head trying to keep you safe by telling you what could go wrong, why you definitely shouldn't do it *that* way and the reasons that, whatever it is, it's going to be a complete and utter disaster. And then, finding other totally unrelated things to add to the argument about why you should or shouldn't do it, giving you more unnecessary things to feel anxious about and stopping you from doing what you know deep down you need to do.

Yep, *that* voice. Your very own podcast of doom, playing on a loop all day long.

But here's the thing. Life is way too short to be spent stuck in unhelpful thought patterns, constantly wrestling with difficult emotions which are taking you away from doing things that will create the life you want. Having a life you love is not just for the very lucky – I believe it is your absolute birthright! And it's entirely possible to have that lovely life if you learn some techniques to quieten the chatter in your mind whenever the overthinking starts up.

life is way <u>too</u> <u>short</u> to be spent
stuck in <u>unhelpful</u> thought patterns!

All of us have that anxious parent popping up from time to time. Sometimes we're able to ignore it, and sometimes we can't (and sometimes we shouldn't, for good reason). The problem-solving safety machine that is our mind isn't trying to make our lives hell, it just loves to do its job well, and we can thank it for that. However, the overthinking can spill over into something unhealthy and potentially damaging – rumination.

Ruminate (v.), from Latin *ruminatus*, 'to chew the cud'

When we ruminate, we are unable to stop the negative thoughts, the dwelling on failure or the repetition of criticisms and bad memories. We replay these distressing thoughts and memories over and over in an attempt to protect ourselves from the negative experiences happening again, while flooding our minds and bodies with the same uncomfortable emotions and reactions we experienced at the time of the original event. In severe cases it can lead to anxiety disorders and depression, and at a minimum we lose hours, days, even months doing it.

If you're prone to rumination, you've probably noticed that it can easily become a routine. You start off with one 'what if?' and you end up in a sort of analysis paralysis that feels uncontrollable – and the more habitual our thinking, the more difficult it is to break free.

The ability to unhook yourself from these thoughts and redirect your attention to something more helpful and meaningful while working to calm and centre yourself is the most powerful way to escape its clutches.

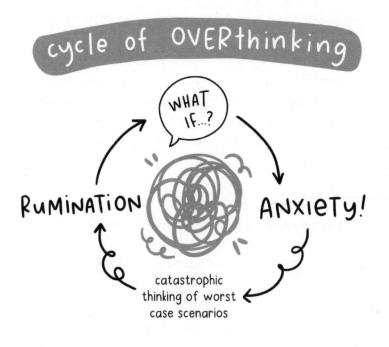

What being an overthinker feels like . . .

- Your mind is constantly racing and you find it difficult to focus on anything other than your racing thoughts.

- You find it difficult to let things go (especially if they're not entirely positive) and don't feel settled until you get to the bottom of why someone said what they said.
- You avoid social engagements or events because you keep replaying embarrassing moments from the past and fear they will happen again.
- You struggle to make decisions, even the ones that feel so simple.
- You can't take risks that lead you in the direction of growth because you always fear the worst.
- You have a hard time relaxing or getting to sleep at night because you can't shut your brain off.
- You feel emotionally drained by your thoughts to the point where you can't feel happy and confident as you go through your day.
- You try everything to stop or slow these thoughts, but they just keep playing in your head.

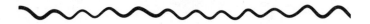

Why do people overthink?

None of our internal organs are there to make our insides cosy; they all have a function. The brain is no different – it looks for problems to solve, and it does that by acting like a time machine. In any given moment, it can grab something from the past and pair it with something from the present in order to interpret what's happening now or will happen in the future. Why? So you can take the best course of action to keep yourself safe.

But this process can get a little trickier if we've had a series of stressful and difficult experiences at any point, an invalidating or unsafe environment growing up, or a traumatic experience as a child or as an adult. These experiences can subconsciously create and shape our deep-rooted core beliefs about ourselves, the world and our future. Our core beliefs are like glasses. They help us see and understand the world more clearly, except, for some of us, those glasses were created from trauma and stress – a critical or unhappy parent, a jealous bully, or perhaps an aggressive and emotionally dysregulated PE teacher.

Unfortunately for us, these negative interactions and experiences formed the foundation of who we 'think' we are and how we believe others to be. They essentially formed the lenses that we see and interpret the world through today, as well as our ideas about how well we can cope within it. If feeling unsafe or criticism, rejection, abandonment, invalidation (I could go on) was an issue for you back then, it's likely your glasses will be on the lookout for it today, in order to protect you from feeling that again. And this starts with a whole bunch of 'what if?'s.

One unhelpful thought leads to another – and they find their friends, their cousins, their sisters and all the other Negative Nancys confirming the negative core belief we already hold. That's how it works for most of us who over-think. You might start off tormenting yourself about a tricky conversation you had with a colleague and, before you know it, you're stuck in your head, agonizing over an incident when you were seven years old that left you feeling embarrassed and rejected, instead of taking action and doing what you need to do to make the current day a success.

A big waste of time, yes, but as you can see, it probably comes from a place you had no control over, so be kind to yourself in this moment, please.

Don't get me wrong – we need the ability to plan and prepare for danger so we can survive it. Thinking deeply and thoroughly is a good way to work through decision-making. But when it becomes overthinking, or rumination, and doesn't offer any solutions, that can lead to worry. And with worry comes anxiety. If you're also a highly sensitive person, you're going to have even more things to process (processing things deeply in our 'thing'), and if you're anything like I was, you're going to have to strap yourself in, as you could be stuck there for hours.

Yes, you may come up with more angles and subtle nuances that others don't, but that usually comes with a price of paralysis by doubt and indecision. Aka, all thinking, no action.

REFLECTION EXERCISE

Have a think about the following questions.

What might your mind be trying to protect you from?
What might your mind be trying to prepare you for?

Most overthinking begins with wanting to avoid a potentially negative or uncomfortable feeling or feeling a need to take control because of discomfort with uncertainty. Humans hate uncertainty! And some of us would rather imagine a negative outcome than not know the outcome at all. So what do we do? We think about the 101 different negative outcomes that could happen so we don't get caught off guard.

Except the 101 negative outcomes never happen. The scenarios you've created in your mind aren't real, but the time you've wasted and the anxiety you feel as a result very much are.

When these unhelpful thoughts come up, we usually do two things. We either get hooked by them, believe them to be true, give them our full attention and obey. Or we try to avoid or escape them by forcing ourselves not to think about it. Let me tell you, either response is ineffective and leads to more discomfort in the long run. If we automatically believe unhelpful thoughts to be true, without looking at the evidence, it will probably take us away from our goals, and if we try to force ourselves not to think about something, we will almost certainly think about it more. Remember our pink elephant from earlier on?

Now, you'd think that the anxiety that comes from overthinking and worry would stop us from doing it, but no. It's just so damn seductive because it's reinforced by all the times you've overthought or worried about something and nothing bad happened. So, if something went well (or, at a minimum, didn't blow up in your face), your mind will subconsciously pair that success to the worrying you did about it beforehand. Now you're so hooked by jumping down the rabbit hole of overthinking and worry that when you *don't* do it, you feel anxious. On top of that, the other unhelpful bonus of being stuck in our heads worrying and overthinking is that it distracts us from the anxiety we feel in our bodies, which, let's be honest, can be worse.

The truth is, you can't stop unhelpful thoughts. But you can stop yourself from getting hooked by them. As Professor Steve Hayes (the Acceptance and Commitment Therapy founder) says: 'There's no delete button in the brain. You can't delete old neural pathways, you can't delete unwanted thoughts and feelings, but what you can do is lay down new neuronal pathways so that when the old ones are triggered, these new ones can fire up and give you a new way of responding so you can unhook yourself from these thoughts and do something different.'

The rest of this chapter will teach you how to do that.

What's the function of your overthinking?

Strange question, I know. But once we can establish the function, we can see if it's worth doing or if there are any other more efficient ways to meet your goal. The common reasons I hear in my practice are: 'It helps me prepare and plan for the worst' and: 'It helps me understand why.'

Have a go yourself – why do you worry?

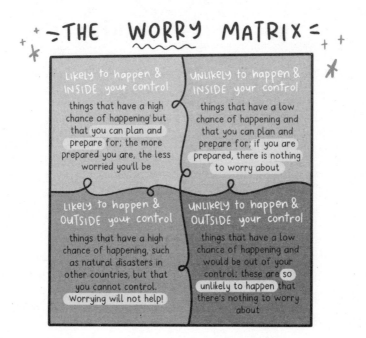

THE WORRY MATRIX

Likely to happen & INSIDE your control

things that have a high chance of happening but that you can plan and prepare for; the more prepared you are, the less worried you'll be

Unlikely to happen & INSIDE your control

things that have a low chance of happening and that you can plan and prepare for; if you are prepared, there is nothing to worry about

Likely to happen & OUTSIDE your control

things that have a high chance of happening, such as natural disasters in other countries, but that you cannot control. Worrying will not help!

Unlikely to happen & OUTSIDE your control

things that have a low chance of happening and would be out of your control; these are so unlikely to happen that there's nothing to worry about

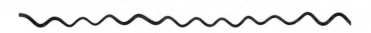

Let's think about the pros and cons of your overthinking. I'd like you to write this down on the grid on the next page – I've started you off with some examples above.

Pro of overthinking: *Deciding a course of action prepares me for the worst.*

Con of overthinking: *It wastes my time and energy.*

Pro of not overthinking: *I can get on with other, more fulfilling activities.*

Con of not overthinking: *I feel less in control.*

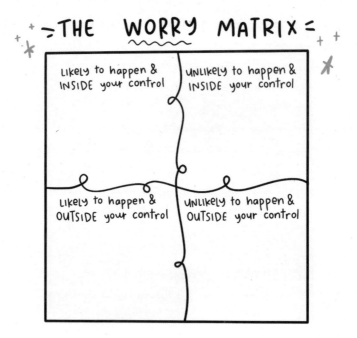

THE WORRY MATRIX

LIKELY to happen &
INSIDE your control

UNLIKELY to happen &
INSIDE your control

LIKELY to happen &
OUTSIDE your control

UNLIKELY to happen &
OUTSIDE your control

If you completed your matrix, then you probably established that, yes, there are some real short-term positives of overthinking, *but* it's not really helping you to show up in the way you want or helping you to reach your end game in the long term. The positives just don't outweigh the negatives.

If I'm right, then I'm hoping that will spur you on to try something different so you can redirect your attention and energy to the things that do. So . . . am I right? Probably. Drinks all round, you're halfway there. Let's do this. I'm going to break this up into six core processes.

1. Acknowledge that it's going to be hard

When you try to change the behaviour of overthinking and worry (yes, it's a behaviour) to something more efficient, your mind may get quite militant and demand that you spend time worrying about this or else something awful will happen, and you may feel a strong pull to listen and obey. Be ready for this. Acknowledge what's happening, thank your mind for trying to keep you safe, sit with the anxiety (it's an emotion you know well, and it won't hurt you) and do what you need to do anyway.

* acknowledge what's happening, * *
thank your mind for trying to keep you safe,
* SIT with the anxiety *
* and do what you need to do ANYWAY!

In these moments it helps to remind yourself of all the things you could be doing if you weren't spending time agonizing, worrying and overthinking.

2. Unhook and refocus

When the thoughts try to grab you – and they will try – it's helpful to use some good old ACT defusion techniques. The simplest one is noticing what's happening and naming it in a non-judgemental way:

'I'm noticing that my mind is trying to keep me safe by telling me . . .'

'I'm having worries that . . .'
'Here is my mind telling me about bad things that
   are going to happen . . .'
'Here is my mind catastrophizing . . .'
'I just had the thought that . . .'

3. Stay present

Imagine if you were able to notice every time your brain was taking you down that rabbit hole of overthinking and could bring it back. You would be more present in everything you were doing – at work, with your partner, your kids, your friends. You'd retain more information, as well as being clearer about how those things made you feel. And it's good to know that so you know what to do more – or less – of. This is mindfulness. It's not something you can master overnight, but it's something you can do at any given moment to refocus your attention back to things that serve you well.

I'm going to be real with you. If your mind isn't used to being still, then at times doing mindfulness can feel hard and unproductive, and doubly hard if you find it difficult to spend any time really being aware of how things feel inside your body. That's all the more reason to do it. Start off with one minute of mindfulness practice per day and double it every day from there.

REFLECTION EXERCISE

If you're anything like me, you definitely want to spend your time doing things that you actually care about instead of what your anxiety tells you. You also want to have a laugh with and enjoy the people you love instead of with your inner critic. If I'm right, get your pen and paper out and have a go at answering the following reflection questions from Dr Russ Harris.

If I waved a magic wand so these thoughts aren't hooking and controlling you:

> What would you stop doing or start doing, do more of, or less of?
> Who would you be more attentive to or present with?
> What goals would you pursue?
> What activities would you start or restart?
> What people, places, events, activities, challenges would you approach, start, resume or contact, rather than avoid or withdraw from?

Think of the brain like any other muscle – it needs to be engaged and strengthened, and regular exercise will make it stronger over time. That's basically what mindfulness practice is – a work-out for your attention (we covered some of this in the previous chapters).

think of the brain like any other muscle, it
★ needs to be engaged & STRENGTHENED ✷
✷ & regular exercise will make it STRONGER
over time!   ★   *

First, you notice when you've been distracted. Then you redirect your attention back. Then you let the thoughts come and let them go, all while sustaining your full attention on something neutral like your breathing, or the feel of the soap suds when you're washing the dishes, or (if you hate doing dishes like me) the feel of the dishwasher tablets as you pop them in the little holder thing, or the sounds around you. That is mindfulness. It's allowing our thoughts to be present in our mind, whether positive or negative, and then choosing to anchor our full attention elsewhere.

We're not trying to achieve perfect, infinitely sustained attention. It's more about the ability to draw your attention back to the present any time you want, no matter how often your mind decides to go on a wander. The more frequently you do this, the quicker you will notice when your mind has gone down the rabbit hole, and the quicker you will be able to pull it back out again.

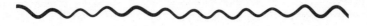

Five ways to use mindfulness when the overthinking starts

- Take ninety seconds to notice your breath; its pace and how the air feels in your lungs and the inside of your nostrils.
- Anchor your attention to any sounds you can hear in the room; see if you can notice different layers to the sounds.

- Put on some fun music and pay attention to any sensations that arise in your body; try to locate where in your body those sensations are (we spend a lot of time trying to avoid sensations in our bodies, and that's half the issue).
- Take a slow stretch and notice any feelings you have in your body, any aches, pains, kinks, any good feeling you get from stretching. Be curious about it, but non-judgemental.
- Focus your attention on the front and back of your hand; see if you can notice anything new, any patterns, any roughness or smoothness. Again, leave judgement off the table.

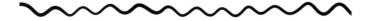

Some people feel they can't do mindfulness because they're always distracted. Well, yes, that's because your brain *works*! It's meant to distract you. We have at least 6,000 thoughts every day – being mindful just means noticing when we're distracted and bringing our attention back. If you've been distracted fifty times and you've noticed fifty times, cool! You have aced it. That's the win!

As long as you keep noticing *when* you're distracted and bring your focus back, you will find yourself in control of your attention rather than the other way around.

4. Time-boxing your thoughts

This is going to sound seriously weird, but hear me out. Overthinking, as you probably know, can happen at any place, any time. Sometimes you're going to be aware of the triggers, but a lot of the time you won't be and so, when it starts, it can very easily interfere with your day-to-day life. One very powerful way to deal with this is to postpone your overthinking to a particular period, effectively putting a box around it and moving it to a specific place and time and for a certain duration each day. When you learn to postpone worry and overthinking, it ends up being less intrusive in your life and you'll be managing your worries efficiently, which is going to leave you feeling more in control. This approach, just like mindfulness, takes patience, so you must be prepared to practise it repeatedly by following these steps.

Create your period to overthink

That's a time, a place and the duration, and it will be the same each day. For example: 7 p.m., kitchen, twenty-five minutes. This place should be free from distractions, and it also needs to be unique. So if you sit in the living-room armchair regularly, then don't make that your rumination place – it must be somewhere you assign purely for the overthinking time.

Postpone your thoughts throughout the day

OK, this is the hardest part. Every time you notice yourself overthinking that's not during your allotted overthinking period, you're going to postpone it. Give yourself permission to think about this thing . . . just not now. Briefly write down what you're overthinking about so you remember it (and I mean super-briefly, in only a couple of words), either in a little notebook or in the notes section in your phone.

Use your mindfulness skills to focus your attention on the present moment

This is where everything we have discussed in this chapter and previous ones comes into play, and it's so important to use these skills.

Think about the most important and best thing you could do for yourself right now

That might be something practical or positive, pleasant or active, nurturing – whatever it is, how can you meet one of your needs right now, while you're waiting for your overthinking period?

Come back to your thoughts at your designated rumination time

Get settled at the place you planned and take some time to reflect on the thoughts you've written down from the day. If some or all the thoughts are no longer bothering you, leave it there – you don't need to do anything else. If you do need to think about them, spend no longer than the amount of time you specified for your overthinking period. Think away to your heart's content, but not for a minute longer than you've allowed for.

5. Problem-solve the right way

It shouldn't come as any surprise to you to hear that over-thinking is not the same as problem-solving. To reduce your overall day-to-day worry, you need the right skills to be able to meet your problems head on, rather than over-thinking or worrying about them.

Problem-solving allows us to tackle issues in the right way. It's constructive, helpful and healthy. It refocuses us on the problem at hand, helps us to devise effective methods for solving it and gives us a clear way forward.

This all might seem simple, but when we're anxious, our ability to problem-solve diminishes, so it's always good to have a foolproof technique or structure to problem-solving at hand. There are two simple questions to help with this:

- Are you concerned about something that is real?
- Are you likely to encounter this problem in the near future?

If the answer is yes to both of these, then you can go right ahead with the six steps of problem-solving, and this is what you're going to be doing in your overthinking period.

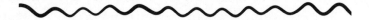

The six steps to problem-solving

1. **Identify the problem**
   Where does your problem come from? What are you aiming to get out of solving it? Is it a problem that we can actually do something about? (let's be honest,

sometimes we create problems in our minds that either aren't problems at all, or problems that we have no control over).

2. **Brainstorm potential solutions**

   Think of a number of possible solutions, even if they seem silly. Ask yourself what values you want to live by as you deal with it. What would you have to change to make this problem no longer a problem?

3. **Consider the short- and long-term implications of your top solutions**

   Look at the short and long-term ramifications or consequences of each of the strategies you've come up with in relation to your wellbeing, your relationships and personal growth opportunities.

4. **Make a choice**

   If none of them jumps out at you, ask a new question – which of these is the least bad? And if you still can't decide, that's a choice in itself. It just means that the problem never gets solved. Move on.

5. **Take action**

   This is the most important step. You're going to put the effort into overcoming the problem. You might need some additional motivation, but it's worth it.

6. **Evaluate your results**

   You've come up with the solutions, you've weighed up the pros and cons of each one, you've chosen one to go ahead with and you've carried it out. Was your plan effective? Did you act in line with your values? Has the problem gone, or is it still hanging around? If the problem still exists, can you repeat the same plan? Or do you need to carry out a new one? If the results weren't great, you might want to go back to step 2. If the results are good but the problem is still there, then you could maybe try repeating steps 3 to 5 before evaluating again.

The key here is to take problem-solving action in line with your values and your end game and, if you can't do that in the moment, focus your attention back to other meaningful things until you can.

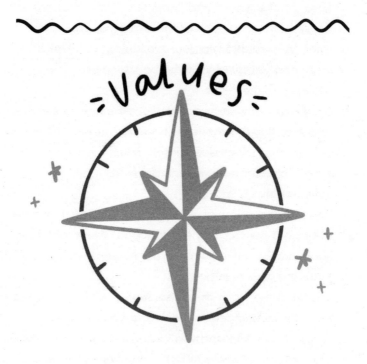

6. Use your values to help you make decisions

Your core values can act as your compass point, making it easier to know exactly what to do and how to show up in tricky situations. Think of it as a mental shortcut. For example, if your top core value is discipline, then whenever you're up against a difficult choice and you find yourself stuck overthinking, ask yourself: 'What action brings me closer to showing discipline?'

Maybe that means you have to set a boundary with a colleague when your anxiety tells you not to, or maybe you have to get yourself to the gym when it's raining. The action to take might not always be easy, but if it's measured against your values, it will be clear. Consistently aligning your behaviour with your values helps you to cut through the noise in your mind and take action to get you closer to your end game. If you need to, revisit Chapter 1, on the Five-part Model, to refresh your core values.

Why is overthinking common for HSPs?

For many HSPs, deep thinking is an absolute strength in both their personal and professional lives. When thinking abstractly, we're able to create beautiful pieces of work. If we are focused more concretely on solutions, we can use deep thinking to explore and analyse every aspect, from the big picture down to the smallest details.

when thinking ABSTRACTLY, we're able to create BEAUTIFUL pieces of work

However, deep thinking can easily turn into overthinking. While our focus flows, it may get stuck on irrelevant details or become unable to settle on a single thought. This can make it difficult to think clearly and arrive at decisions. Our mind may be on a clear path towards a solution, but overthinking could cause us to start questioning ourselves, possibly even bringing out our inner critic to send us on a spiral of negativity and self-judgement.

Ideally, you'll begin to recognize these common patterns faced by HSPs so you can work to manage them. And as you learn to identify the signs of overthinking, you can use that awareness to lead yourself towards more intentional decision-making. A good place to start is to list some decisions that are easy for you to make and some that are particularly difficult. What is the difference between these types of decisions? What makes one easier than the other? Are there more difficult emotions like sadness or fear attached to harder decisions; are your thoughts more positive or negative? Do you have more practical resources at your disposal when you find it easier to make decisions?

The power of thoughts

If you watch a scary movie, you're going to be frightened, even though it's on the TV or a cinema screen. Likewise, the movie in your head when you're worrying about different catastrophic scenarios has an impact on you, and probably not a good one. So let's flip it round and use the power of thought to lead you in the direction of something that *doesn't* make you feel dreadful.

It doesn't even need to be positive – mindfulness is just about being neutral and noticing every kind of thought with no judgement. We want to get to a place where you say: 'Oh, I just had the thought that [insert unhelpful thought here], but I'm going to focus on my breathing and anchor myself instead of completely tying myself to it.'

Use mundane tasks to practise mindfulness – washing the dishes, packing the dishwasher (cough, cough) or drinking a cup of tea can both be done mindfully. You just need to use as many of your senses as you can to anchor your attention. The more you do that, the quicker you'll be able to notice when your mind has drifted off and bring it back and, soon enough, it'll be like clockwork.

This is where neuroplasticity comes in again (we talked about this in Chapter 1, on the Five-part Model) so we can create new pathways in our brain enabling us to do different things and get different results. Through repetition, we're honing that skill and carving out a more streamlined way to focus. Every time we do it, we're getting rid of the old pathways and creating new ones which

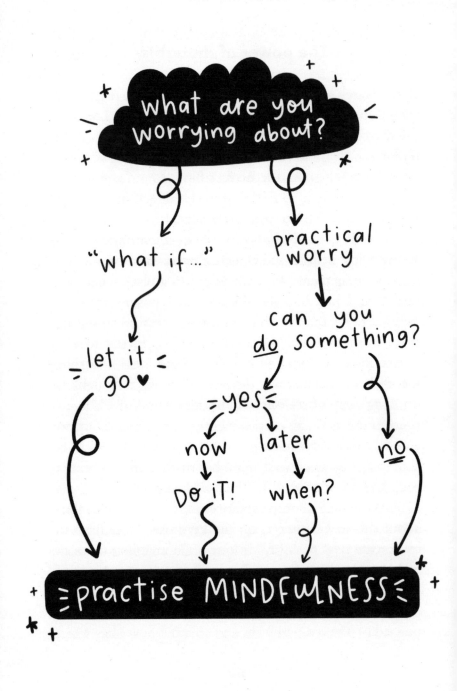

make it easier for us to get to the present moment. I feel so excited when I think about the potential for all of us to retrain our brains. Practise every day, remove judgement, and you'll see that some of these things that have gripped you gradually start to unravel.

Overthinking at night

When people come to my clinic, before we even start talking about all the stuff that's going wrong with them, I check how much sleep they're getting, how much water they're drinking, how much food they're eating and how often they're moving their bodies. We can cut out a lot of the excess stress and distress by making sure we get those things on point from the off.

If we haven't slept well or enough, we're not as equipped to deal with stress and we're basically setting ourselves up for failure. Thanks to social media and society's obsession with the hustle-hustle culture, a lot of people have this 'I'll sleep when I'm dead' approach to life. Um, are you a robot? I think not. And so, like every other human, you need sleep – around eight hours or so a night – and that should be a priority over all else. Honestly, sometimes it just comes down to sleep. Sleeping is a healing process, so allow yourself to heal; if you sleep well, you will feel more ready to face the day.

sleeping is a HEALING process so allow yourself to heal and you will feel more READY to face the day

But to sleep you need to be relaxed, and if you're over-thinking and feeling anxious about the day, that's not gonna happen. Anxiety being manageable during the day then coming in like a ton of bricks once you're winding down at night is a super-common experience. For a lot of us, being at home in the evening is the first time we've been alone with our thoughts. I know what it's like – you're in your bed, all cosied up, away from the stress of the world and – *bam!* – your brain lights up and finds itself ruminating about every worry that you managed to hold off during the day. Bye-bye, sleep.

Ironically, sleep deprivation can be a trigger for anxiety during the day. So you're now in a vicious cycle in which anxiety can cause sleep deprivation, and sleep deprivation influences anxiety. I mean, how cruel is that?

You don't need me to tell you that this is just not sus-tainable. The only way to break this cycle and get a good night's sleep is to combat the overthinking and worrying that creates the anxiety. It helps to start preparing yourself for sleep hours before you hit the hay so, once you're in bed, that's when you can draw your focus on calming your mind and body.

Develop a sleep routine

Sometimes it's not actually the overthinking that stops you from getting to bed on time – when you've been so busy during the day, your late evening might be the only time you have to yourself. And so you find yourself in this revenge bedtime procrastination, where you put off sleep to claim your personal time back and make the most of your evening – aka scrolling on Instagram and Pinterest until 1 a.m. looking for new kitchen design ideas.

I get it, but that's not sustainable either – sleep must be prioritized. Having a wind-down routine can help your body transition from day to night. Don't do anything that's overstimulating, like scrolling through social media or binge-watching *Bridgerton*. Instead, make your routine calming and quiet with down-regulation activities that trigger the relaxation response such as mindfulness meditation, stretching, yoga or deep breathing. Then deliberately spend time 'feeling into' the resulting good sensations in your body, signalling to your brain that it's time to rest.

Go to bed and wake up at the same time every day, even at weekends

The body and mind love consistency. Going to bed and waking up at the same time every day follows your body's natural circadian rhythm – or your internal clock. When you get up and go to bed at different hours, it disrupts this rhythm.

Create a relaxing environment without distractions (especially from blue lights on your devices)

If you must have a TV or computer in your room, avoid using it before going to sleep. In a nutshell, the blue light from the screen deceives your body into thinking it's day-time and slows the release of melatonin, the hormone that helps us relax and fall asleep. Charge your phone in a different room and put it on flight mode. Organize your sleeping space to keep it clean and clutter-free so you're not overthinking about how messy it is.

Get some sun

Getting some sun on your skin during the day is directly linked to your quality of sleep. Go outside, away from the artificial lights indoors, two to three times a day if you can, and plan for times when you can spend the entire day outdoors.

Learn to be present

Mindfulness changes the way we perceive and respond to our thoughts. Rather than going down a negative spiral of thoughts, practise observing them and then allow them to pass. Consider listening to a meditation app like *Headspace* or do a deep-breathing exercise on your own.

No caffeine after 1 p.m.

Caffeine blocks the sleep-promoting chemical adenosine which is produced in the brain when we are awake. That means no coffee, no tea, no cola!

Pencil in some downtime

For many of us, getting into bed is the first time we've stopped and pondered on our day. So, rather than jumping into bed after a long, stressful day, set aside some time to process everything that happened before you go to sleep. Jot down any worries or stresses on a piece of paper if you need to. Whatever you do, don't use this time to do anxiety-inducing tasks like paying bills or catching up on work emails.

Limit napping – or avoid it altogether if you can

Taking cheeky naps during the day disrupts your circadian rhythm, making it harder to fall asleep later and making you more prone to waking up during the night. Try to stop it altogether, but if you really do need to nap, keep it to thirty minutes or less and avoid napping later in the afternoon.

Use your bedroom only for sleep

If you work on your laptop or watch TV in bed, your mind will start to associate each of those activities with being alert, focused and awake. If you can't get to sleep within thirty minutes, get up and read a boring book. When you feel yourself getting tired, go back to bed. This pattern teaches your mind that your bed is meant only for sleep. Over time, you'll naturally feel more tired when you lie down, and it'll make it easier to fall asleep.

Something worth thinking about . . .

Worries about worries, and worries about thoughts all maintain the act of worry as a whole. If you're playing a past scenario over in your mind, there needs to be a point to it. Rewriting the script in your mind is not helpful unless you're doing it to inform how you want to behave in the future.

Sometimes people say they worry because they think they're going to miss something if they don't. If giving that problem your attention actually helps, then let's do that properly and solve it. You *know* that most of the things you worry about don't happen. And the things you continue to worry about? Well, you're still alive, so it looks like you're able to handle it! At some point you have to start looking back with perspective, trusting yourself to make good decisions and having the confidence that you can manage whatever life throws at you.

You've got this.

at some point you have to start looking back with perspective, TRUSTING yourself to make good decisions and having the CONFIDENCE that you can manage.

CHAPTER FIVE

Imposter Syndrome

'When I won the Oscar, I thought it was a fluke. I thought everybody would find out, and they'd take it back. They'd come to my house, knocking on the door: "Excuse me, we meant to give that to someone else. That was going to Meryl Streep."'

– Jodie Foster, on winning the Academy Award for Best Actress in 1989 for The Accused

we can
UNDO our
imposter
stories

A question for you. Apart from all being total goddesses, what do Beyoncé, Michelle Obama and Serena Williams have in common? It might come as a surprise, given how phenomenally talented, successful and positively badass they are, but all three women suffer or have suffered from imposter syndrome. So if you too are plagued by self-doubt, convinced that your every accomplishment is a fluke, and live in fear that any minute you're going to get found out and exposed as a fraud, then at least you're in good company . . .

Imposter syndrome totally gripped me while I studied for my doctorate in clinical psychology. I was the only black person on the course (there were two in the next cohort – an improvement, I guess) – I walked in on the first day and three quarters of the class were blonde females with posh accents. Am I exaggerating? Perhaps, but it definitely felt that way.

So I, with my long braids and hybrid south London street/Cockney accent, understandably felt different and immediately questioned if I was really meant to be there. I thought that everyone else was really smart (I mean, next-level smart) and they seemed to be breezing through all the assignments while I felt I didn't know what I was doing. Academically, I'm OK. I went to a normal comp in Lewisham – not exactly the world's best school – and only scraped a 2:1 at uni, and that backdrop set the tone, because my imposter syndrome has never been more acute or apparent than when I was doing this doctorate, surrounded by people who seemed to be worlds apart from everything I knew.

I didn't necessarily find the work super-hard, but I struggled to articulate my answers to questions in class. Nobody there was from the same place as me, nobody looked like me, they all hung around together and, although no one was ever mean, I found it very difficult to fit in. I was from Catford. I didn't have horses or fields. I was trying to be a different version of myself, and it was exhausting.

They would invite me out for drinks, but I couldn't bring myself to go because I knew it would be hard work for me to try and keep up with their conversations about their skiing trips. *Too* hard. I felt completely out of my depth and that I had nothing to add to the conversation. In the end, I'd deliberately come late to class to avoid having to make small talk. I was officially fused with the imposter story in my mind, and that impacted how people saw me.

I remember thinking that people had low expectations of me, as if they were surprised when I got a good grade (I always got good grades in the end; that's part of the deception of imposter syndrome), but I guess they only ever saw me being very quiet and chill, coming to class late and rarely contributing, so why *wouldn't* they assume I was hopeless? The imposter syndrome didn't stop me doing the work and ultimately getting my doctorate, but it made things infinitely harder for me because the doubt in my ability to get it right would bring on procrastination. This meant everything was lastminute.com, which would lead into guilt and anxiety because I'd put everything off for so long. And then into over-functioning and overworking to make up for it. It was an exhausting vicious cycle.

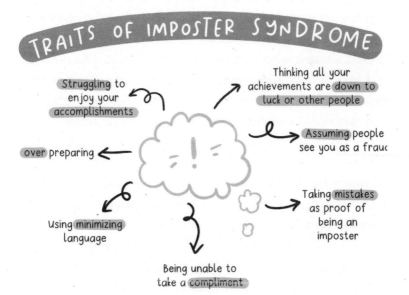

TRAITS OF IMPOSTER SYNDROME

Struggling to enjoy your accomplishments

Thinking all your achievements are down to luck or other people

over preparing

Assuming people see you as a frauc

Using minimizing language

Taking mistakes as proof of being an imposter

Being unable to take a compliment

What is imposter syndrome?

People who experience imposter syndrome find it difficult, if not impossible, to accept their own achievements. They feel inadequate and incompetent, and the crippling self-doubt is compounded by a persistent fear of being exposed as a fraud. Not surprisingly, imposter syndrome disproportionately affects high-achieving people, leaving them questioning whether they deserve what they have accomplished. The concept was originally called 'imposter phenomenon' by its creators, psychologists Pauline Rose Clance and Suzanne Imes, who did a study in 1978 that focused on high-achieving women and wrote: 'Despite outstanding academic and professional accomplishments, women who experience the imposter phenomenon persist in believing that they are really not bright and have fooled anyone who thinks otherwise.'*

I don't know about you, but for me there was this feeling that this house (my career) was one built on sand and that it could get washed away at any moment and leave me there naked in front of everyone (yes, I'm dramatic). And for women in particular, this feeling can be a large contributing factor to a general lack of confidence. The battle to keep up appearances can lead to perfectionism (we'll cover that in depth in the next chapter), holding yourself back because you feel too useless to progress and hating being part of a team because group situations leave you vulnerable to being 'found out'.

You tell yourself that if you just make sure you always produce ten-out-of-ten work and never put a foot wrong, then everything will be cool; no one will ever know it's all

* Pauline Rose Clance and Suzanne Imes (1978), 'The imposter phenomenon in high-achieving women: dynamics and therapeutic intervention', *Psychotherapy Theory, Research and Practice*, 15 (3).

a fluke. If you do everything on point, then people won't realize you're a fraud. Sound like a recipe for disaster? Of course it does, because that's exactly what it is! Not only does it give rise to all the over-functioning, but it's also physically impossible to be perfect a hundred per cent of the time, so you're setting yourself up to fail.

it's physically IMPOSSIBLE to be perfect 100% of the time so you're setting yourself up to fail!

Imposter syndrome doesn't just affect people in the workplace, it can impact your relationships, too. FFS, I know. You get some success on Bumble, but you can't unhook from the imposter story that this person is only staying with you because they feel too guilty to leave – it could never be because they actually want *you*. But here's where it gets juicy: that insecurity is going to influence your behaviour – needing constant reassurance about the status of the relationship, being too clingy or too distant will of course affect the other person, and not in a good way, and you'll end up with the type of relationship you don't want at all.

There are other psychological difficulties associated with IS, such as feelings of shame, guilt that you've 'duped' people, anxiety, stress, fear and even depression. The whole shebang. And highly sensitive people are particularly susceptible because, with all that fine-tuned thinking, there are so many more stimuli for us to draw on and add as evidence that we shouldn't be here.

In short, imposter syndrome can stop you from taking chances and moving forward in your career and your life, and we need to stop that. Are you with me? Good.

> *imposter syndrome can stop you from taking chances & moving FORWARD in your career & life... we need to STOP that. *

Tell me your imposter story

If you're dealing with this right now, the first thing you need to do is acknowledge the imposter story that's got you hooked. The content of your story probably includes lots of doubt about yourself and your abilities, with a sprinkle of 'I shouldn't be here.' Then you reframe that story – use the actual evidence of your situation to create a more balanced and realistic story. If you're in a good position in your career, remind yourself of all the qualities you have which got you there, all the work you put in to achieve what you have. If you're fused with your imposter story like I was, then it's very likely that it's clouding your judgement and so it might be helpful to find a friend or someone you trust to help you look objectively at what you've achieved and how you've achieved it. I mean, just go and have a look at your CV and, if you really drill into the detail, you'll find that 'luck' rarely has anything to do with it.

This process of gathering evidence against your imposter story will, in turn, change how you feel about yourself, which will change your behaviour and motivate you to take your foot off the brake, put it on the gas and move in the direction of growth.

Wherever you are, you deserve to be there. And with a little intent, you will soon start to feel like the confident, capable, intelligent and qualified superstar you undoubtedly are.

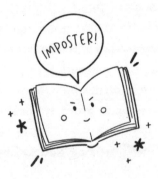

REFLECTION EXERCISE

Take some time to think about the following questions.

What's your imposter story?
When does it show up?
What type of situations trigger it?
What does it sound like?
What stories does it tell you when it's triggered?
What does it feel like?

What emotions does it bring up for you?
How does it make you behave?
What does it stop you doing or make you do too
    much of?

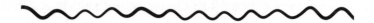

Why are successful women more prone to imposter syndrome?

- Despite education and training, they feel unable to break self-doubt.
- They feel pressure to be a good 'role model'.
- The workplace culture is competitive and there is intense pressure to succeed.
- There are more men in senior leadership roles, so women feel a need to prove themselves.

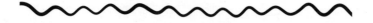

Where it stems from

As adults, we are products of our experiences, and so the triggers for imposter syndrome can go all the way back to childhood. If you have brothers and sisters and were always divided up as 'the sporty sibling', or 'the academic sibling', or 'the creative sibling', as you get older and end up doing things outside that mould, you might end up feeling that you shouldn't be.

But research shows that the biggest contributing factor to imposter syndrome is discrimination. If you're in a minority, whether that's to do with ethnicity, sex, disability or any other protected characteristic, and you go to a place where you don't see yourself, you're going to question whether it's somewhere you should be. That is standard. There are about seven black psychologists in the whole of the NHS. I'm joking, I'm joking, there are more of us than that, but we are very thin on the ground.

You don't even need to be treated differently by anyone. If you're in an environment where the other people are mostly things you are not, then it's instinctive to wonder if this is the place for you. The messages you're getting are that people like you are not in jobs like this, therefore it must be a fluke. It couldn't *possibly* be because you're good at what you're doing! It must be some sort of diversity quota, or a mistake, or a sneaking in via the back door-type situation.

We're going to talk a lot more about comparison a little later in the book, but that's the instant feeling we get when we see a room full of what we are not. If we already have limiting beliefs about ourselves and they are coupled with limited representation, we're going to lean into the imposter syndrome. Again, we're looking for everything in line with our negative core beliefs and discounting anything that says we're not an imposter. You're taking that comparison and using it as evidence that you're a phoney, and it's scuppering your chances of the progression I know you are more than capable of.

if we ALREADY have limiting beliefs about ourselves & they are coupled with limited REPRESENTATION, we're going to lean into the imposter syndrome. ✳

⋗CASE STUDY⋖

Louisa starts a new job in the City. She arrives on her first day and it's immediately clear to her that she's different to most of her colleagues. Whereas Louisa went to a state comprehensive, the vast majority of her co-workers have been privately educated, and many of them have connections which go way back.

They seem supremely confident and knowledgeable, and she feels excluded, uneducated and not worthy. They discuss subjects she doesn't feel informed about. These guys fit the mould.

Louisa retreats. She gets her head down and does the work but contributes very little, if anything at all, outside of that. She assumes that whatever she says won't be good enough so it's better to keep schtum. She doesn't ask questions, she doesn't join in the conversations, and this knocks into other areas of her life as well, including her general self-esteem. Louisa gets used to being the person who doesn't speak up.

*

Louisa's situation might sound familiar to a lot of you, whether it relates to university or a workplace or any other setting where you've felt like a fish out of water. But we can undo our imposter stories. If Louisa made the decision to ignore her imposter voice, taking it slowly by speaking up occasionally and building up to contributing more frequently, she would probably find that the imposter story became less and less real.

When the imposter story starts playing, Louisa needs to ask herself whether those thoughts and the feelings they trigger are really something she needs to act on. Remember, we're not trying to get rid of the emotions, we're just sitting with them, giving them some attention and possibly leaning into them to see if there is anything we need to solve.

> + we're not trying to get rid of the *
> emotions, we're just sitting with them, +
> giving them some ATTENTION & possibly
> * leaning into them to see if there is
> + + anything we need to solve +

Women and the social contract

Research has shown that imposter syndrome disproportionately affects women, and it's not hard to see why that would be the case. The higher women climb up the professional ladder, the less we see ourselves represented and, for many years, by the time we reached boardroom level, we were virtually non-existent.

There are signs that things are changing now (about time too, right?), but Pauline Rose Clarence and Suzanne Imes found that women suffer from imposter syndrome more frequently and more intensely than men because of the Western social constructs that bind us all. From the day we are born and then throughout our years growing up, we are all – men and women – subject to conditioning, and an unwritten social contract sets out and tailors very clear roles for and to us.

So, girls are 'told' we're going to be mothers, wives, homemakers, caregivers and sometimes that's all we're going to do. That's our thing. The men go out and make the money. As women, we might make *some* money, but the big bucks come from the men. We all take part in this contract unconsciously, but these beliefs are so ingrained, so deepseated, that it means women have lower expectations for success. And so, when we *do* become a high achiever, we believe we're a fraud who must have got lucky.

Getting to a point where you're stepping outside all those rules often doesn't feel safe. You can still do it, especially if you have good support behind you, but it can bring on some anxiety because you are breaking that social contract.

Yep, you're right: the contract sucks. And these so-called rules? We need to smash them. Women are here, and we need to gas each other up to stay here. And that means we all have to be conscious of the ways we might be unwittingly reinforcing the 'rules' – things like making our little girls wear cute shoes with bows in the playground instead of trainers, which means they can't run and jump and play like the boys. Or deliberately dressing in a 'typically' masculine way (hello, power suit), not because that's how you feel comfortable but because you think you won't get taken seriously if you wear a dress. Whatever you're wearing right now – that is your power suit because *you* are in it!

I guess, because we're new to this and it's only in the last couple of generations that it's been the norm for women to work full time, we're still playing by the rules that have always been there. That is a hundred per cent going to change because there are women the world over – I've got people in my programme who are up at 3 a.m. in Australia for our coaching sessions – who are determined to rip up that rulebook.

Trust me, it's happening. Things will be better for the next generation, thanks to the bright, brilliant women currently paving the way. We can all contribute to and take a piece of the pie.

Change the narrative – find your passion for compassion

People with imposter syndrome will take every blip as proof that they don't deserve to be there. They will start talking to themselves very unkindly, oblivious to the fact that in doing so they're putting themselves back into threat-response mode.

When our emotions are up and we're experiencing anger,

sadness and anxiety, our judgement becomes clouded and we're not thinking clearly or coherently enough to solve this setback efficiently. So first, we need to make sure that we're talking to ourselves with compassion.

When you're feeling down about yourself, along comes the negative mental filter and – you know the drill – it's going to take you away from where you need to be. If we're talking to ourselves negatively, then that's going to bring on uncomfortable emotions which will lead to actions based on those uncomfortable emotions. And if that's the case, our actions are usually not going to take us in a direction we want to go.

We can make things much easier for ourselves by getting back into problem-solving mode and asking: 'How can I turn this around?' Practise humility, embrace failure as a part of success and not the opposite of it and, most of all, stop striving for perfection. It's a losing game and not a worthy one.

You're going to find your compassionate voice and it needs to do its thing.

REFLECTION EXERCISE

We're going to find your compassionate 'other'. This could be something like a spirit guide – even an imaginary monkey guru. Whoever or whatever it is, it's going to help you through this by leading with kindness, wisdom and empathy.

What does your compassionate other look like? What does it sound like? What is the tone? What are the words it uses?

Sometimes people imagine another person, an angel, a rock, a fairy godmother, a tree. I've even had a client imagine it as an elephant.

Imagine the colours and the aura and step into that.

Whatever you need to hear and see at the times you're feeling like an imposter, conjure up this compassionate other and it will help you recover some balance.

Getting rid of the imposter story

I can't lie, the imposter story is hard to shift, especially if this has been a long-standing thing you've had every single time you've gone into a new job or undergone some sort of transition. But what keeps that story relevant is all the behaviours you do in order to avoid being found out. Those behaviours reinforce the idea that, yes, you *are* an imposter and you are going to get sussed.

As you do the exercises in this chapter, your imposter story is going to tell you, 'But this doesn't apply to you, you actually *are* an imposter, so don't bother!' so you need to remind yourself that it's just a story.

If it feels like a fact, it means that you've been hooked by it, good and proper. Now you need to work on getting yourself unhooked. Remember we talked about singing unhelpful thoughts to the tune of 'Happy Birthday'? You can do that to unhook yourself from imposter syndrome (*The Addams Family* theme tune is another good one). It feels silly, but that's the point! Try it now. Find one of your common IS thoughts – maybe it's 'I'm such a fraud' – and see if you can sing it out.

However, the quickest way to shut down the imposter story is to make sure your actions are the *opposite* of what it tells you about yourself. If you didn't feel like you were an imposter, how would you be showing up differently? If you felt like you were meant to be here, how would you be showing up differently?

In short – what does someone who is not an imposter act like? Do that.

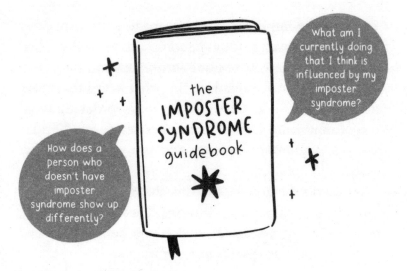

Changing the behaviour

Your behaviour needs to be in line with someone who thinks they deserve to be there. It's going to be hard because difficult emotions will be triggered and your thoughts are going to tell you it's ridiculous, you're kidding yourself and it's all a lie. But you are now officially your own biggest cheerleader, so you must cheer yourself to victory. Encourage yourself, keep that compassionate, non-judgemental and super-wise voice in your back pocket and take the wins to build your confidence.

For example, if someone gives you a compliment – accept it. Get really good at receiving positive feedback. Collect it, and see how it feels to actually take it on board rather than downplay it. It might not fit in with the narrative you have of yourself, but just say thank you! Appreciate it! Even if it's for the sake of the other person and allowing them to feel good.

Maybe your confidence has only gone from two to two and a half out of ten. Next time it might go to three. They are all little wins, and you build it up while moving forward and reinforcing the shiny new beliefs you want to have about yourself.

* * get really good at receiving POSITIVE * *
* feedback. Collect it & see how it feels *
to actually take it on board rather than *
* * downplay it!
  +

How I'm beating my own imposter syndrome

Even after I'd qualified, the imposter syndrome lingered. I'd be introduced to people – 'Meet Michaela, she's a doctor' – and get all stressed because now I had to appear smart when sometimes it felt like I couldn't even string a sentence together! I didn't like being in a position where people had expectations of me, because I felt incapable of meeting those expectations.

However, it rears its head less and less frequently these days. That's the result of getting (and accepting) positive reinforcement from my time in the NHS. This turbo-charged my belief that I *was* meant to be there after all. Every time I got positive feedback from a client or a supportive email from my manager, I would screenshot it and save it in a folder on my phone. This helped me massively. Every time I started to notice the IS story, I rummaged through my phone and brought up actual evidence that the story just wasn't true.

I accepted that I wasn't good at what I do because of a diversity quota, luck or over-functioning. It was actually about something that was intrinsic to me: my highly sensitive trait, my willingness to learn and my drive. I'm going to toot my own horn and tell you that I was easily engaging with clients my colleagues who'd been in the game for years struggled to work with ('Send Michaela!' became a familiar call).

More than anything, I saw that my authentic self was

what clients connected to. And I wasn't doing anything extra special; I was being myself, talking to real people as if they were real people.

Getting results through therapeutic relationships quickly became my strength. I kept putting one foot in front of the other, working with more and more 'hard to reach' and 'hard to engage' clients and, soon enough, there was no evidence for the imposter story and I felt comfortable at the level I'd reached.

When I left the NHS to move into private practice, my clinic quickly became full and my clients frequently referred their friends and family, which was further validation. I was able to do this on my own. I was officially good at my job.

I'm kind to myself at all costs, but my imposter story is rarely kind, so I don't give it any energy or attention, and for good reason. If I hadn't ignored it, I wouldn't have gained the evidence I have now that confirms that it is truly just a story. I don't know if my IS will ever be completely 'cured' because I'm continuously doing new things and the triggers of not seeing people who look like me are always going to be there. But it comes and it goes again. I don't allow it to stop me or change anything. And I certainly don't lean into the thoughts that tell me this means I'm not meant to be here.

If I did, I wouldn't have the Instagram page and I certainly wouldn't be writing this book!

CHAPTER SIX

People-Pleasing

'Don't be afraid of losing people,
be afraid of losing yourself trying
to please everyone around you.'

Saying YES to everything is creating an EXPECTATION you're going to have to spend the rest of your life TRYING to fulfil... & THAT is a sure-fire path to BURN-OUT!

I'm a people-pleaser at heart and have been since child-hood. I was a very quiet kid; I never complained when someone upset me and I always did as I was told. I got my homework done without having to be nagged and once even devised a detailed schedule for my parents to follow in the mornings so I could please, please, PLEASE, be on time for school every day.

Great for my parents and my teachers, but for me it was all underpinned by the fear of getting into trouble and the inevitable shame that would come with that. That's what I was trying to avoid. I hated the spotlight being on me and I wanted to dodge that at all costs.

I felt I needed to appease people so I could steer clear of any potential conflict which might change how people viewed me (yep, even as a child), and I carried this through with me into adulthood and the workplace, right to the point where shit got real.

There's so much more to being a people-pleaser than just showing others the odd bit of kindness. Of course, making people feel happy is not a bad thing, but we must be very clear about where our generosity is coming from.

If it's crossing a line into something problematic to us, then we're gonna need to scale this right back. Being worthy in other people's eyes only because of what you can do for them is never an ideal situation. We're not here for that.

Later on in this chapter I'm going to talk about what happened when my own house of cards came tumbling down, how being a 'yes (wo)man' risks burn-out and the importance of setting boundaries and learning the art of saying no, which will free up more time to do what *you* want to do. I know that you want to create a life that keeps you feeling good about yourself. You want to get that sense of enjoyment and mastery from the things you do, as opposed to doing all the extra tasks that aren't in line with your values, purely because you feel pressured or obligated.

I can assure you that finding your voice and using it to say no, unashamedly and unapologetically, is going to be life-changing.

+ I can assure you that finding your voice
★ & using it to say no, unashamedly & ★
+ UNAPOLOGETICALLY, is going to be +
life-changing! ★ +

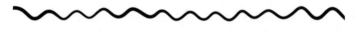

Traits of a people-pleaser

- Don't think highly of yourself
- Need others to like you
- Need validation

- Can't say no
- Over-explain yourself
- Apologize or accept blame even when it's not your fault
- Quick to agree
- Struggle with authenticity
- Give, give, give
- Have next to no free time
- Have a fear of conflict, even if it's nothing to do with you

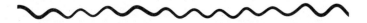

Inside the mind of a people-pleaser

If you thought that at your core you were a capable, likeable and loveable person, would you feel the need to constantly please others at your own expense? Would you always have to prioritize others over yourself? I'm thinking, no.

Unfortunately for many of us, due to difficult childhoods, traumatic experiences or anything to do with relationships with others that we found hard and struggled to process at the time, we developed negative core beliefs about being unloveable, or just not good enough. For example, if you had a parent that had quite unpredictable moods that felt scary at times, then you may have grown up thinking you had to keep them happy by doing everything they say so you didn't have to feel their wrath. As a result, and in order to protect ourselves from mistreatment, abandonment or rejection, we develop 'rules for living' to compensate for some deficit we think we have.

We have an infinite number of rules about how we live and act which are designed to keep us from feeling how badly we did 'back then'. A common rule for people-pleasers is 'If I do things for others, they will love me and I will be good enough.' Does that resonate with you? If it does, I'm sorry you were made to feel this way. You are likeable, you are loveable, you most certainly are good enough, and you don't need to seek anyone's approval but your own.

♥ you are LIKEABLE, you are LOVEABLE, you
* most certainly are GOOD ENOUGH, & you ♥ *
♥ don't need to seek ANYONE'S approval
♡ but your own. ♡ *

This is why setting boundaries is soooo hard for people-pleasers. The thought of creating conflict and being disliked is very painful, because it feeds into our negative core beliefs, breaks our rules and, as far as we're concerned, that comes at a hefty price. For example, if you think you're not good enough and that it's easy for others not to like you, rather than ending up with no friends and possibly no job either (catastrophic thoughts, yes, but it's hard to be aware of them in the moment). And so you just smile and say yes to everything, agree with every opinion and hope that all will be well because you know you have value, even if you're doing things you don't want to do, showing up in a way you don't want to and leaving little room for you to be your authentic self.

So far, so familiar? Let's continue.

You want to fit in and so you show up as the person who you *think* will get the most 'likes'. The upshot of that is you end up with a group of people who like the fake version of you, and it gets very hard to shift the expectations that come along with that. Sure, you might be attracting people, being that easygoing 'yes (wo)man', but they are potentially the wrong kind.

Now you're in a position where in order to keep your place in the group you have to maintain this inauthenticity, which is hard work, tiring and means you never get to see how anyone responds to your true self.

I have news for you: there is probably a shedload of people who very happily rely on you being a people-pleaser. But we can't necessarily judge the people asking you to do all the things. After all, as far as they're concerned, you're the person who *likes* doing everything! You do it every time! And probably with a smile, too! They're not mind-readers and so we have to forgive them for not knowing you resent it.

When it comes to career and business opportunity, you might have developed a fear of saying no that is compounded by the culture of your workplace. Time and time again I see work environments that encourage overworking, over-functioning and, let's face it, burn-out. It gets to the end of your working day – you know, the point where the company stops paying you – and you decide you're going to leave on time for a change so you can go and enjoy life outside of the office? And your manager, who also struggles with work–life balance, fuelled by their own insecurities, sashays by with their eleventh cup of coffee, unrealistic expectations and a quick 'Oh, leaving already, Annie?', followed by a disapproving side eye.

So now you feel bad and end up staying an extra hour. And to add insult to injury, the same company (after realizing that half their staff are on long-term sick leave) has the audacity to bring coaches in to talk to employees about how *they* need to be more 'resilient' instead of supporting them to create work–life balance *rolls eyes*. With all due respect . . . do one.

When looking at some of what maintains the fear of saying no in the workplace, I like to bring in the concept of scarcity mindset versus abundance mindset. Abundance mindset is when you are confident that the things you desire will continue to flow to you and there's enough of the pie for everyone. Scarcity mindset is when you're fearful that opportunities are going to run out and so you operate on the basis that this is your last or maybe your only chance. If you don't take it, someone else will and it'll be lost for ever. That's good old-fashioned FOMO for you.

But saying no doesn't mean the offers stop. Remember that thing you have that made people want to ask you in the first place? You've still got it! It just means you're able to *choose* to say yes to things that are in line with your values and what's important to you, rather than taking on everything and getting into situations that aren't great for you.

REFLECTION EXERCISE

Why do you struggle to say no? Where does that go back to? What are you trying to protect yourself from?

What emotions would you need to tolerate in order to get better at setting boundaries?

What thoughts would you need to unhook yourself from in order to get better at setting boundaries?

Highly sensitive boundary-setting

It is particularly hard for highly sensitive people to set boundaries. We are constantly absorbing and processing other people's emotions and body language and, if we're already coming from a place of not feeling good enough, then anything we receive back is going to be viewed in line with our negative core beliefs. The high sensitivity makes the build-up to, process of and the responses to setting the boundary – good or bad – feel bigger. And if you know it's coming, then you're going to try and avoid it because it's easier (in the short-term, at least) to just say yes and carry on as you were.

But now we know the negative impact of trying to avoid uncomfortable emotions, right? And we're on a mission to feel any emotion and still show up in the way we need to in order to create a life we love, right? OK, we're on the same page.

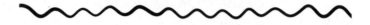

If you tick more than three of the following, then you're probably the office people-pleaser.

- Helping colleagues feels like a full-time job in itself.
- Delegating tasks makes you feel uncomfortable.
- You regularly agree to unreasonable requests.
- You feel unappreciated for all the commitment you give.
- You feel guilty when you don't work beyond your contracted hours.
- You assume it's your fault when things go wrong.

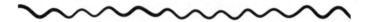

The pitfalls of people-pleasing

A couple of years ago I learned something so mind-blowing that it made me resolve never to worry about setting a boundary again. When people are having an organ transplant, surgeons sometimes give them stress hormones such as cortisol in order to shut down their immune system temporarily so it doesn't reject the new heart or lung.

Let that sink in.

The impact of stress is potentially so huge it can cause your immune system to shut down. And if that's prolonged, then you're opening yourself up to all kinds of health complications and conditions.

That's when I realized this was not something to play with. It's not 'just' stress. If you are in a near-permanent state of threat response, the cortisol is running through your body for way too long and you're doing yourself no favours. Saying yes to everything is creating an expectation you're going to have to spend the rest of your life trying to fulfil. And that is a sure-fire path to burn-out.

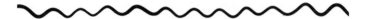

The five tell-tale signs of burn-out

You are emotionally distancing yourself from colleagues

When we're feeling low or sad, we withdraw. In terms of evolution, if you're not seen, you're not going to get hurt or killed. So you hide. And it's easier to opt out than having to find the energy to keep up your inauthentic self.

You are demotivated

Your motivation and interest in many things go down and you no longer feel passionate about your work. This apathy can extend into your everyday life as well, because you're emotionally and physically spent.

People have noticed you're not yourself

You think you're doing everything to hide it, but the nature of burn-out means others will notice that you're not showing up in the way you usually do.

You're getting sick more than usual

There's nothing left in the tank to fight off infection and so any cough, wheeze or bug going round, you're going to pick up. And it could floor you.

You're drained and irritable

When you're full to capacity with uncomfortable emotions, anything on top of that is going to feel unbearable or unmanageable. You're simply not going to have the headspace to regulate your emotions.

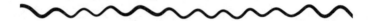

What burn-out feels like

In 2019, the World Health Organization officially recognized burn-out as an 'occupational phenomenon', upgraded from its previous status as a stress syndrome.

This is good! It highlights that the go-go-go attitude in the workplace is not optimal or healthy.

When you're stressed, you can still function and do what you need to do. Having a little bit of anxiety can even get you out of danger and propel you to get the work done. But when you're burnt out, your whole thinking is diminished. Your emotional cup is full. You are tearful, your stress levels are sky high, to the point where anything else is going to tip you over the edge.

It means your emotions are all over the place; your brain is scrambled. You can't focus or function at anything like the rate you were at before.

Burn-out is your body screaming for help. It's saying:

'OK, you don't wanna listen? You knew you were stressed six months ago, and you didn't do anything about it. So, now? Now, there's nothing you can do. Now, every time you wake up to go to work, that is going to be a struggle. And, actually, sometimes you're not going to make it in at all.'

The impact of that amount of constant stress on your body is holistic and can take a long time to recover from. Take my word for it, if you don't slow down now, burn-out will *make* you slow down.

burn-out is your body SCREAMING for help... if you don't slow down now, burn-out will MAKE you slow down.

My own experience came in 2019, when I was working between the NHS and private practice. I started doing the Instagram page as well, which was taking up more of my time, and I got to a level I'd never worked at before and haven't since, simply because I know I can't. And I'm OK with that.

I was forced to become boundaried, which is now one of my core values and one which I refuse to compromise on. I value myself, my health and my sanity too much for that. Now, my biggest stress management technique is simple – figuring out how to cut my 'to-do list' in half. Yes, half! And saying no. It works like magic, let me tell you, and is probably the best starting place for you, too.

REFLECTION EXERCISE

Imagine your child is in front of you. Or your bestie, or the child version of you. They are overworked, overloaded, tired and stressed out. What would you say to them?

You'd probably give them really good advice, advice you desperately wanted them to follow, aka take a frikkin break!!!

As uncomfortable as it feels, give yourself that advice, and take it. Treat it as an experiment if you must, and just see what happens. Do it before you even believe that setting a boundary will be fine or that leaving that piece of work until tomorrow is going to be OK. Just try it, that's all I ask. It's very likely you're overestimating the negative impact of slowing down and underestimating the positive, but you have to follow this through to know for sure.

Window of tolerance

I think now's a good time to introduce you to the concept of the 'window of tolerance', originally developed by Dr Dan Siegel MD, Clinical Professor of Psychiatry, and why chronic stress is a no-no. Your window of tolerance is that perfect level of arousal you need to cope with emotions and function well in everyday life.

Everyone has one and, unfortunately for those who have experienced trauma, the zone of tolerance may be a little narrower than it is for others. This is completely understandable, as you're likely more primed to detect a threat in order to stop it repeating. In this case, even small stressors can cause anxiety, irritation or anger and lead you into what's called states of 'hyper-' or 'hypo' arousal. If this is you, then please remember, hold compassionate space for yourself and take judgement off the table.

You are doing the best you can and working to change things for yourself. You are winning.

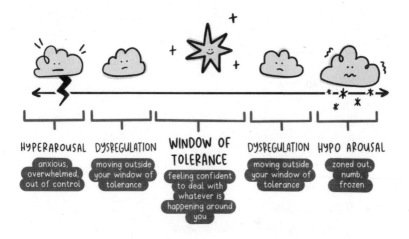

Hyper- and hypo arousal

Hyperarousal is a heightened state of activation or energy also known as the 'fight or flight' response. We discussed this back in Chapter 3. If you're in this mode, it means your nervous system is on high alert and probably triggered by 'perceived' threat (whether or not there is real danger doesn't matter), or traumatic memories.

You basically have too little arousal because your parasympathetic nervous system (which we also talked about previously) has been overloaded. This can impact your appetite and your sleep, make you stay away from socializing, mean that you struggle to talk about how you feel and you end up feeling emotionally numb.

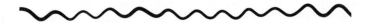

Hyperarousal symptoms include:

- Angry outbursts
- Fear
- Anxiety
- Emotional overwhelm
- Panic
- Hypervigilance
- Tight muscles
- 'Deer in the headlights' freeze

Source: NICABM (2021)

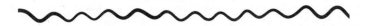

Hypo arousal, on the other hand, is essentially the opposite. There's more to it than that, but the detail can get quite confusing. We know it as the 'shutdown' or 'freeze' response and it can be triggered by the same things as hyperarousal, such as chronic stress, feeling threatened or remembering traumatic events.

If you feel like you're stuck 'on', if you struggle with sleep and concentration, always feel tense and have the occasional (or frequent) angry or hostile outburst, you could be experiencing hypo arousal.

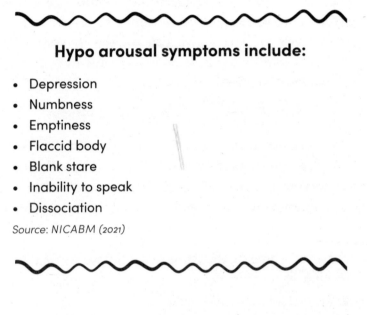

Hypo arousal symptoms include:

- Depression
- Numbness
- Emptiness
- Flaccid body
- Blank stare
- Inability to speak
- Dissociation

Source: NICABM (2021)

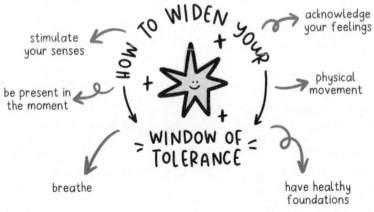

How to widen your window

Life is hard a lot of the time, and even if we're the best at setting boundaries and managing our time, being 'successful' in the Western world means being able to tolerate certain levels of stress. We can do this by essentially broadening our window of tolerance and looking after our nervous system.

Recognize what it feels like when you're experiencing emotions outside of your tolerable zone.

Take it a step further and honour your nervous system by putting pen to paper and words to feelings. Trust me, your nervous system will benefit from your attention and your awareness of what state it's in. As a start, you can write down the following:

What are some of the day-to-day difficulties that typically overwhelm your nervous system?
How does it make you feel?
How does it impact your body?
Rate your level of hyper- or hypo arousal from zero to ten (it's actually a good idea to do this periodically throughout the day – in your head is fine).

Physical movement
This can be small or big – standing up, brisk walking, switching chairs, marching on the spot or star jumps – and is especially useful for coming back from hypo arousal. Yoga

is incredible for getting you back into your window of tolerance; it's the perfect balance between rest, present moment focus and effort.

Have the right foundations in place

If your sleep is poor, you aren't fuelling your body with nutritious food and you're not exercising, or if you have unchecked physical pain or illness or substance misuse, then it's likely your window of tolerance will be narrower.

Ground yourself to the present moment to create feelings of safety

For example, say out loud to yourself: 'I'm in my office, it's 28 May, I'm with my colleagues, I'm safe.' You could even imagine being in a safe or calm place. Close your eyes and use your five senses to describe what it looks like, how the air or temperature feels on your skin, what you can smell, and even what you can taste. Maybe your safe place is on the beach with a daiquiri in hand . . . I'll see you there!

Stimulate your senses

Smell is the fastest way to the thinking brain, so reach for your fave scent. Find some chewy, crunchy food, roll a pen between your palms, get a stress ball or go and wash your hands and give yourself a little hand massage while you're there. Try feeling the soles of your feet on the floor or your bum sitting on a chair.

Use your breath to anchor to the present and your body

Remember, we spend a lot of time trying to avoid our bodily sensations, and that is part of the problem, so try slow, deep belly-breathing, with a longer exhale. Count your exhales and find places where you feel your breath moving in your body, for example your chest, abdomen or throat. Place a hand on two of these places and feel the breath moving between both of your hands. Then add a mantra to repeat on every exhale.

Setting boundaries

I'm going to let you in on a little secret. Most people aren't even going to be aware you're setting a boundary. I mean, feel free to announce it if you wish, but it really doesn't need to be a big deal if you don't want it to be.

Sometimes we can give off the impression that we believe we're not good enough, and certain people will jump on that, play on it and use it to their advantage. But if we're saying no with a smile (just as we used to say yes with one) and staying in line with our values by leaving the person making the request feeling good, then we're giving out messages about who we are with every interaction.

People will come to expect that you will help them if you can but that you won't take a project on if you have too much else to do. This is the goal. We're doing this for us, and people will understand that we are worthy of being treated well. Why? Because we treat ourselves well.

I set a boundary myself just recently. I had a master-class which I had said was going to be delivered on a certain day, and there were 15,000 people on the email list waiting for it. But I was swamped. The only way I could have got it done would have been by working through the night, and I really didn't want to do that. Something had to give, and so I held my hands up.

I sent an email to everyone on the list, around 12,000 people, and explained that I'd made a promise to myself not to go back to 2019, when I was trying to do everything and making myself ill because of that. I said, in this instance, I was going to lead by example and put the master-class out two days later than planned so I could get it done to the level I wanted it at and not dig myself an early grave in the process.

So many people came back and thanked me for being honest and leading by example. They said that was what they needed to hear and, if *I* was able to say no to all of these people, then that showed them that they could too! I wasn't just telling them no; I was showing them how it's done.

Now, fulfilling my promises is a value of mine. But Acceptance and Commitment Therapy tells us that values are like a cube – in any position, some faces are visible and some are not. One value might be very important in that moment, while the others are in the shadows. So I want to fulfil my obligations, but I also want to be boundaried, and so I gave people an understanding of the reality. Yes, I had feelings of guilt, but guilt is just that – a feeling – and I knew I'd be fine if I just sat with it and allowed it to pass. As long as I didn't give my attention to the thoughts that were creating the feelings of guilt in the first place, I knew I'd be good. Emotions only last around 90 seconds anyway. It's the rumination that prolongs it.

Giving your authentic self creates trust, connection and communication. When you are raw and real and tell people the truth, how can they argue with that? There are going to be some people who aren't going to enjoy you finally setting some boundaries and, well, you have to be prepared for that. But, you know, that can be enlightening in itself if it's going to give you an insight into the people around you. Who is getting your attention and energy? Should they be?

giving your AUTHENTIC self creates TRUST, connection & COMMUNICATION.

If you can't put in a reasonable boundary that is important for your mental health and wellbeing without consequences, then you need to reconsider how much attention this person gets from you.

They may not be right for you, and that might be a tough pill to swallow, but it is what it is. They're going to have to deal with that, and you don't need to absorb their feelings. Acknowledge, but don't absorb, and that will help you create distance. You're probably thinking, 'Don't absorb others' feelings? Yeah, right. Easier said than done.' I get it – and what follows should help in the moment.

- Acknowledge that you feel 'something'.
- Name the feeling.

- Confirm with yourself that the feeling isn't yours.
- Bring your attention to the part of your body where you feel the most calm and focus your attention there – even if it's just your nose.
- Visualize a light beam going from the top of your head all the way down to your feet and clearing out the other person's emotions.

In any event, I'd wager that you're letting your imagination run away, thinking about the 'catastrophe' that could result from putting in a boundary, as well as underestimating your ability to cope with any feelings that arise from the conflict it causes. There are probably a few people in your life right now that you need to set clearer boundaries with. You wouldn't be reading this book otherwise. All I can say to that is: 'There's no time like the present'. Do the damn thing.

REFLECTION EXERCISE

Go back to the values you identified in Chapter 1, on the Five-part Model. Think about how you can stay in line with these values even when one appears to be in conflict with another. So you might want to be supportive and helpful but also boundaried. How can we inject that supportiveness into our 'no' without making our behaviour the problem?

This might look like giving the person a compliment about the project they're working on and leaving them feeling good about themselves. But you're still saying no.

The art of saying no

The reality of saying no is often far more mundane and non-consequential than you ever imagine it to be, especially if you tap into what's important to you while you're doing it. This person is asking you to do something because they trust that you're going to do a good job, so let's lean into that. Show gratitude, but also be very clear around the fact that you can't do it.

I'll even give you some templates to make sure you get it done! These are from personal experience and the amazing book *F*uk no!* by Sarah Knight (Thank me later.)

To a colleague or someone pitching you an idea that you just don't have the time for:

'I'm really grateful you thought of me for this, but because of my schedule I can't commit to it right now. I wish you all the best with it.'

To your boss asking you to take on additional work:

'That sounds like a great project. My caseload/workload/to-do list is really full at the moment, so please let me know what you would like me to prioritize' (or, even better, 'Please let me know what you would like me to put aside for the moment so I can allocate my time).'

To a friend who asks you to help her move house when you are working to an important deadline:

'I hope all the moving preparations are going well. I can't help tomorrow because I have a big deadline at work. I can come over to the new place for a couple of hours and help you unpack on Saturday, though. Excited for your big move!'

To your sibling (or anyone) who asks to borrow money:

'I wish I could help you with this. I've had a look at my finances and it's just not going to be possible. Let's get together on Friday and think about other ways we can work it out.'

To a friend who invites you to come and join a group activity, but it sounds boring and you really can't be bothered:

'That's not really my scene, so please go ahead without me and enjoy! Let's get a date in the diary for us to meet soon, though. I'm free on——. What about you?'

Don't apologize. Don't say 'unfortunately'. You don't even have to say 'because', depending on who the person is. There's no need to over-explain, because that reinforces the idea to yourself that simply asserting your boundaries and needs isn't good enough.

If you're saying, 'I can't do this,' why do you need to give people more than that? You can of course be vulnerable if you want to show that, but gauge who needs to hear or see that vulnerability.

The vast majority of people will respond positively to this very clear no and say it's fine and thank you for letting them know. However, if you're an overthinker and/or a highly sensitive person, I know for a fact you're now sitting there, thinking: 'What if they don't really mean it?' That's where your mindfulness can come in.

Take people as they are. You are doubting their response. How about you doubt your doubt? That's what you need to question, not the person receiving your kind and gracious no.

What definitely *isn't* an option is not responding at all, so let's take that off the table.

By ignoring the other person, we are turning our pain into suffering because now we also have the worry that we haven't got back to them. Sure, saying no feels awkward to you, but we can feel uncomfortable emotions and we can do hard things, so close that box as soon as you can by facing the initial discomfort and doing what you know you need to do. The more you do it, and the more you exert that boundary, the further you will reinforce the idea that you are worthy of saying no and the world doesn't end just because you aren't doing something someone else asked you to.

This is communication, this is life. So let's give off a vibration to the world that isn't fuelled by the negative thoughts we have of ourselves. Let's not lead with this any more, let's not say yes when we want to say no. The knock-on impact is just not worth it.

And you never know who is watching. It might be someone who is going through the same thing and is inspired by your ability to say no unapologetically but also with love and kindness.

Self-destruction versus self-care

After all these years of putting yourself last, it's high time you switched up your priorities. We hear a lot about 'self-care', and that is all well and good, but it has to be more than taking a bubble bath once in a while.

Let's make looking after ourselves a regular thing from this day onwards (you will have more time now you've started saying no!) and ensure *your* self-care is as luxurious, as opulent and as extra as you can afford. Yeah, the money could go elsewhere, but this is a prescription – it's what the doctor (me!) has ordered. So, take a whole day off, go for afternoon tea with your friends, pop into that shop where they do the bath bombs, put the eucalyptus leaves in the bathroom and dive in.

If you're not used to putting yourself first, there will be discomfort, there will be guilt. Guilt feels absolutely awful, and for good reason, but it's likely that your 'guilt' is based on your negative core beliefs rather than anything you're actually doing wrong, so don't let it knock you off track. Remember, if we want to break the unhealthy rules that

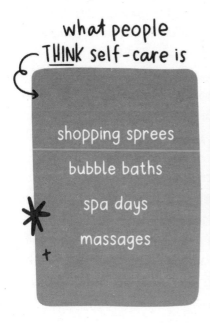

what people
THINK self-care is

shopping sprees

bubble baths

spa days

massages

what self-care
ACTUALLY is

boundaries

saying no

exercising

mindfulness

healthy eating

positive self-talk

we've created for ourselves, then we can't just talk about it, we actually have to break the rules.

Accept the guilt, sit with it, but still look after yourself. You need to show yourself every single day that you are worthy of being looked after, you are someone who cares about and takes care of themselves. You put effort into you.

Taking care of your body with regular fresh air, sleep, exercise, nutritious food and water is also part of this. We've already talked about the transactional relationship between our gut and our mood, but there are foods that can affect our hormones, trigger intolerances or make us sluggish and irritable. And all of that is contributing to our ability to handle day-to-day stresses.

I always recommend clients with anxiety or low mood to go to the GP to get their bloods checked over because sometimes there's a bunch of non psychological stuff contributing. For example, there might be a thyroid issue going on, hormonal deficiencies or a lack of vitamin D. It can also be worth getting an intolerance test – if you're eating things that are causing inflammation in your gut, this is going to be sending signals all around your body that will impact your mood in a negative way.

Make sure you're getting regular exercise because, without it, you're robbing your body of the hormones that are going to keep your mood afloat and your mind full of that sense of mastery and achievement. Some people actually get enjoyment from going to the gym. I would love to be that person but, dear reader, I am not. Instead, I see it as medicine. If this is also you, anchor your motivation around health and mood rather than body image or which person on Instagram you want to look like.

If you can't face the gym, try a mindful walk. I know how cringe that sounds. Back in the day, if someone had told me to go on a mindful walk, I'd be like: 'Err, no! Are you all right?!' But all it really involves is walking around, looking at nice things, being present and switching off from the stresses and thoughts that are keeping you anxious.

Come on, trees and squirrels sound fun, right?

When you have those uncomfortable feelings running the show and think you don't deserve to be looked after, someone telling you to have a day to yourself is an alien concept. I understand that.

But just try it. All the people you think are going to miss out because you're putting yourself first for a change? The opposite is true. Your partner is going to get the happier version of you, your children, too, and your colleagues. Step into that scenario in your mind – does that feel better than the current situation?

Well, you can get there. You may not feel that you are worthy or good enough, but at some point you're going to have to act as if you do. And that's not 'fake it till you make it', by the way, because this is how you've decided you want to show up and all you're doing is stepping in line with that.

So it's not fake, you're finally just doing what's meaningful to you.

Be a boundary-setting bad B

None of us started our careers with the intention of being burnt out and unhappy. That is not what life is about. Success shouldn't come at the expense of your inner peace.

I've got a clear focus for myself now, so it's very easy for me to see what I can and can't say yes to. That is all tied into a bigger picture of helping and supporting people and, in order for me to *give*, I need to be solid within myself, not stretched completely thin. Trying to pour from the empty cup is nonsense. I don't wanna give people little dregs of cold coffee. I want to give them the hot, sweet and plentiful tea, and I can't do that if I'm drained and empty.

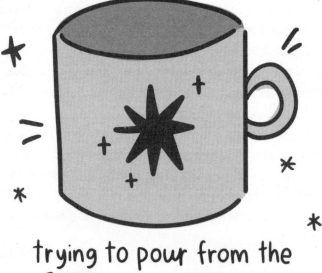

trying to pour from the EMPTY cup is NONSENSE

You've got a clear choice here. You can either stop this by suffering a catastrophic burn-out which leaves you needing meds just to get out of bed. Or you can stop it by starting to say: 'Thank you, but I can't commit to that.'

The benefits of setting those boundaries and saying no are indescribable, and you'll feel instant relief and empowerment, encouragement and reinforcement. All you need to do is make that 'no'-shaped leap and you'll be a boundary-setting badass who won't look back.

Go on, jump!

CHAPTER SEVEN
Fear of Failure

'There is freedom waiting for you, on the
breezes of the sky. And you ask, "What if I fall?"
Oh, but my darling, "What if you fly?"'

– Erin Hanson

you're

overestimating

the threat of FAILURE &

underestimating

your ABILITY to handle it.

If you're striving for perfection in everything you do, then I'm sorry to be the bearer of bad news, but you're chasing the impossible. You're never going to feel like you've achieved it.

What is a perfect thing anyway? Is it possible to take a 'perfect' shower? Can you *actually* make the 'perfect' spaghetti Bolognese? You see, not everything can be 'perfect' and certainly not a hundred per cent consistently, so defining yourself by being a 'perfect person' and basing your entire self-worth on that is laying the groundwork for all of the 'failure' you fear. Every. Single. Time.

And let's say you *did* fail. Why does the idea of that make you feel so bad? That's not a trick question, by the way – you might have to dig deep to find the answer, but once we've peeled back some layers and had a root around, we might get closer to the core belief you have about yourself that makes perfect seem necessary and failure seem like torture.

My guess? You have an intense fear of failure because . . . wait for it . . . you just don't feel good enough and you never have. Perfectionism is a rule you've created to protect yourself from failure and the distress that comes with it. It's basically a defence mechanism. If you felt you were good enough, then, whatever happened, you would be compassionate to yourself and, if it hadn't worked out quite as you'd hoped, you would try again. You wouldn't feel the constant urge to compare yourself to others either.

perfectionism is a rule you've created ✶
to **PROTECT** yourself from FAILURE & the ⁺
⁺ ✶ distress that comes with it ✶ ⁺
⁺

The fear that arises with the thought of failure exists at such a level because it taps into a core belief, and that's extremely painful for you. If you don't do well on this paper, or excel in the baking contest, or create the most magnificent fancy-dress costume the kids have ever seen a) you think that people are going to judge you negatively and that's going to hurt and b) you know your core belief of not being good enough is going to rush up, and that's also going to hurt. You'll probably avoid situations which could poke those negative core beliefs (I bet procrastination could be your middle name) because, if you don't try, you can't fail, right? And not trying and failing because you tapped out is less painful than trying your best and failing. But, when you don't try, you don't give yourself the chance to see that you *can* do this and it will be fine. Whatever the outcome. Damn, you might even enjoy it!

But instead, your fear of failure is taking all those possibilities off the table as well as preventing you from getting rid of the fear itself. Failure becomes this huge monster on a pedestal that you're sure will gobble you up with shame if you reach it. So instead, you just stay away by any means necessary.

No one feels confident a hundred per cent of the time. What you *can* feel confident in is your ability to get through this. You can cope. Keep that in the back of your mind and it will propel you forward because, at the moment, you're overestimating the threat of failure and underestimating your ability to handle it.

But remember: you've been through shit. You have never been more equipped to deal with anything than you are right now. When your mind is stuck on anxious thoughts and worry, cut to the chase and ask yourself what's the worst that could happen if you just went for it? Then ask yourself what practical steps you would take in that event.

Great, now you know that, whatever the outcome is, you can deal with it. Let your thoughts pass, unclench your jaw, put your shoulders down, breathe deeply and slowly, stay present, remember your end game and do what you know you need to do.

Signs that fear of failure could be holding you back

- You hesitate to get involved with new things.
- You procrastinate a lot.
- You spend a lot of time dwelling on mistakes.

- You undermine your successes and don't believe in yourself.
- You engage in negative self-talk.
- You are settling for less than you deserve.

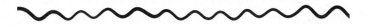

When perfectionism becomes toxic

Every perfectionist I work with has super-high, rigid standards – some are so unrealistically high that they can only be met at a great cost, if at all. Usually, their self-worth is based on the ability to meet these unreasonable standards and, when they are not met, they won't say: 'OK, that was a little unrealistic. I did my best, though – after all, I'm not a robot.' Oh no, no, no. They will settle on: 'I failed, I just didn't work hard enough,' and then they'll try even harder.

And, if they *do* meet a standard, will they bask in glory of the achievement? Not for very long. If you're anything like I was, this is the part where imposter syndrome comes in and tells you: 'It was a fluke' or: 'It was an easy thing to do anyway.' Give me a frickin' break, please.

What do we perfectionists do in order to keep up with these high standards? We focus our attention on the things we aren't achieving in the way we would like so we can correct it: repeatedly checking work for mistakes, excessively organizing, making a million to-do lists, constantly correcting ourselves and others, giving up quickly, avoiding tasks we think we won't be able to do to our standard, waiting to the last minute before doing a task, struggling to make decisions.

These behaviours may protect you from failure, but they take up a lot of time and probably take you away from showing up how you want to. They maintain black-and-white, all-or-nothing thinking and stop you from proving to yourself that your perfectionist beliefs just aren't true.

Now, don't get me wrong, I love a bit of conscientiousness. Wanting to do a job well should be applauded and, if your diligence and attention to detail aren't causing you or anyone else a problem, that's fine. Don't change it. I'm not here to tell you to alter something that has no negative impact on your life.

However, there's a line. If you feel like your need to get everything done perfectly is making you procrastinate, or spend ridiculous amounts of time going over and over the same things again and again, or if it's making you feel super-anxious and affecting your ability to complete the task on time, or driving you to actions that are having a negative impact on your life, then those are all signals that it's becoming toxic. And this is something we need to address.

Tying the success of anything to your own self-worth and only wanting to do a good job because it's underlined by the rule that it must be done perfectly, otherwise you're a failure, is when perfectionism crosses the line into something potentially harmful. It's also very difficult to break free from, because when you're a person who does a good job every time, you're going to get chosen to do stuff! And the positive responses you get from all that effort further reinforce the perfectionist in you.

Some people will see anything they don't do really well as failure. If you have an underlying belief that what you're doing is not good enough, then you will see everything through that lens. You might do something which everyone else thinks you've pulled off fantastically, but you only see one little thing that you didn't do, or which went slightly left and so, now, in your eyes, you've failed.

We need to be able to hold on to the positive experiences as much as we're currently holding on to the negatives, if not more. When your whole self-worth is based on a hundred per cent perfection every single time, anything outside of that is going to leave you feeling broken. If you don't practise celebrating and reflecting on the 'well done's and the 'good enough's, then you are constantly going to feel disappointed in yourself. Do you really want that for you?

we need to be able to hold on to the +POSITIVE experiences as much as we're currently holding on to the negatives!

REFLECTION EXERCISE

I want you to take a few minutes and really consider the following questions.

What core beliefs do I have about myself?
Do I truly believe I am worthy of love and success?

Do I need to be perfect in order to receive
approval?
Where did I get the idea that perfect was the only
option for me?
What does a good enough person look like?
What do they do day to day?
How do they show up?

Where your fear comes from

This fear of failure and the expectation of doing everything perfectly very rarely start in adulthood. Ask most
people who are struggling with this, and they'll be able to
trace it all the way back to primary school. It will often
have been held together by a desperate search for approval
from the person who never gave it.

Maybe you had parents who had exceptionally high
expectations because they wanted you to do well. It might
have been drummed into you from a very young age that
to be successful you had to work at 110 per cent all the
time. Perhaps nothing you did was ever quite good enough
in their eyes, even if it was done with the very best of
intentions. They thought that by withholding praise, they
were spurring you on to greater heights.

For any readers who are parents, it's worth reflecting on
the fact that what we don't address in ourselves, we could
risk passing on to our children. It's a tough pill to swallow,
I know, and just trying to keep your kids fed and watered
is hard enough, but if you struggle to address a fear of

failure or any of the issues I talk about in this book for yourself, then make it about something bigger than you and consider doing so for your children. It will make all the difference.

Sometimes it comes from the school, especially if you went somewhere that was competitive and high achieving, where students were constantly ranked and the kids who did really well in maths, English and science got the gold stars.

It's also a societal thing. The hardest workers, the most driven and ambitious, are the ones who are seen as keeping the economy going, and that's something we all benefit from. I don't necessarily agree with the way we judge intelligence and success. For example, the standard IQ tests, while great at identifying working memory, verbal comprehension and reasoning, usually completely ignore human elements such as emotional and moral intelligence. According to an article in *Forbes* magazine in 2012, Albert Einstein's IQ is estimated to have been around 160 and John F. Kennedy's was only 119. It would be great if parents, schools and society as a whole were geared up to lean into our individual strengths and natural creativity and then give us the space to explore all of that.

So, it's no wonder you don't know how to deal with disappointment or failure, because you've probably been running away from it ever since childhood.

The role of trauma in fear of failure

Childhood trauma has a lot to answer for when it comes to fear of failure, and if you're thinking, 'Well, that's not me, I wasn't abused,' then please be clear – childhood trauma isn't just physical or sexual abuse. It's also feeling unseen by your parents so you think you have to perform or act in certain ways to get their love. It's having people constantly invalidating your feelings by telling you what feelings to have or not have, or that you're too sensitive and so now you're hesitant to show certain emotions and struggle to regulate any emotion that doesn't feel good.

It's having a parent who constantly shouts or withdraws affection because they struggle to regulate their own emotions, so now you get into threat mode any time someone gives you a hint of criticism or distance. It's having a parent who doesn't know how to set their own boundaries and so modelled to you how to get taken advantage of, and now this just seems normal.

I repeat, there's no judgement here – we are all products of our environment to a certain extent. Your parents, too. But we have to stay conscious of our wounds, where they come from and the action to take to heal them.

♥ we have to stay CONSCIOUS of our ♥
wounds, where they come from, & the
♥♥ ACTION to take to HEAL them. ♥♥

Destination: procrastination

So, as per usual, you've said yes to everything and now the pressure feels unbearable. You can't face the astronomical workload so you put off tackling it, then put it off some more (and then a bit more) until you're backed into a corner and looking down the barrel of a very imminent deadline.

The motivations behind procrastination vary – you might be putting it off because the work bores you, or it might be down to panic because you've got too much else going on. But, if you're reading this book, it's most likely to also be underpinned by the fear that you're not going to do a good enough job.

You don't want the feeling of not being good enough, or the anxiety, the guilt, and whatever else you envision is going to come up for you when you're doing this piece of work. And that's where the procrastinating comes in – it's enabling you to avoid uncomfortable emotions and thoughts.

Basically, avoidance is besties with procrastination and their cousins are uncomfortable emotions.

Holding so tightly on to this belief that we're not good enough will have a biological impact, too. Our nervous system and brain see any failure to achieve something as a threat to survival and so instead will look to do something else that we know we *can* achieve, whether that's returning something to the shop or watching another episode of *Real Housewives*. It just seems like a quicker and surer bet (and more rewarding in the short term) than that piece of work you're unsure about. Further reinforcing procrastination in itself.

These delay tactics are turning your pain into suffering, because here's the thing: that work still needs to be done and, if you're just kicking the can down the road, that can is eventually going to trip you up. Unless you literally disappear off the face of the earth, you are going to have to deal with it.

Procrastination can also be a form of self-sabotage – we're always looking for information that confirms our negative core beliefs or fears. If you put something off for so long that you end up doing it badly, then that proves what you always thought of yourself anyway, doesn't it?

As soon as you find yourself doing this, ask yourself, which value do you need to be showing in this moment? And which values are you neglecting by showing up in this particular way?

There are some unhelpful positives about procrastination which keep it going. First, you feel relief from avoiding the task, and second, you get pleasure from the things you are doing to procrastinate, whether that's scrolling through social media or cleaning the kitchen. But when looking at the negatives, is it really worth it?

You end up feeling guilty and embarrassed that you haven't done anything, you reinforce your unhelpful rules around perfectionism and failure, you criticize yourself in your mind, which activates your threat response. (All my clients tell me they're just lazy and not cut out for this, and I'm like: 'No! You're just scared.') The work piles up, making you feel anxious and keeping your threat response activated even longer (hello, anxiety).

Not to mention that you might actually fail if you don't

hand anything in and, with the thought of that, your nervous system is buzzing, but here's the gag, if you're anything like I was, then in the back of your mind there's this little devilish voice saying, if you fail because you left it to the last minute that's sooo much better than starting early, trying hard and failing.

All of these compound and end up making the initial task feel like even more of a drain, and procrastination seem like the better option.

✳ ꞊CASE STUDY꞊ ✳

Clarice is a 32-year-old engineer, successful by anyone's standards, but she has been stuck at the same level in her career for the last five years. She has the talent, she has the drive, but she also has the anxious parent in her mind following her around 24/7.

Clarice takes on yet another new project with the hopes of getting noticed for promotion. The deadline is looming, but the only thing she's done up until this point is procrastinate. She thinks she's lazy, not cut out for this, and this is why she hasn't been promoted.

The real reason she's procrastinating is because her manager hasn't given her a proper brief and she genuinely doesn't know how to get started with it.

She could ask her manager for clarity, but Clarice's overthinking mind tells her: 'No, you probably shouldn't email your manager about this because she's too busy and she'll get annoyed and then she'll think you're incompetent. And remember when you were six and asked the teacher to help you with spelling, and she embarrassed you in front of the class by saying you should already know this? And then Becky made fun of you for a week, and you didn't want to go back to school. Remember that? Yeah, don't do it, you don't wanna feel like that again! Just wait, you'll figure it out yourself.'

How to stop procrastinating

I find all sorts of things to procrastinate about; it's such an easy trap to fall into.

The first thing I ask clients who are grappling with this is whether the resources they have right now are enough to get the job done to the standard they want. Sometimes those practicalities are what it boils down to. And if you don't have the resources, how can you go about getting them? If you're struggling to get your head around a task, is there anyone who knows how to do it? Well, ask them.

When you're in threat mode, which often happens when we have a looming deadline, it might be difficult to see that you have a really clear-cut choice here: ask for help and do a better job, or don't and continue to let it eat you up.

Sure, you might have to sit with some uncomfortable thoughts and feelings for a while, and you'll probably worry that the person will think you're not competent, but that's unlikely to be true and, if it is, you can prepare for that.

Take Clarice, our case study. If she had the core belief that she was good enough, then the anxious parent in her mind wouldn't need to step in and save her from cata-strophic consequences and she would have had no issue with asking for help. Disconnecting from the anxious par-ent in her mind would put her in a much better position to take action and get the clarity she needs from her manager so she can complete the project on time, without the anx-iety, and put herself in the running for that promotion.

Try and look at asking for help as a mini challenge within the bigger challenge of getting the work done.

Another thing I always double-check is whether this task you're procrastinating over definitely needs to be done. Not just this week, but ever? If it doesn't, get rid of it. I love taking things off people's to-do lists!

Try writing three headings and put each item on your to-do list under one of them.

1. Must be done or the project goes to sh*t.
2. Would be nice to do it, but there are no real consequences if it's not done.
3. Neither of the above.

Anything under headings 2 or 3 can go.

You could also request that your manager or supervisor, if you have one, helps you to prioritize and/or takes things off your list. After all, they probably gave you the work to do in the first place, and it could be a good way of getting them to see whether or not what they are asking you to do is realistic. Yes, you will have to tell them that your work-load is too high and that might feel uncomfortable, but you can deal with discomfort. Not getting anything done at all because you're burnt out is a whole other level.

OK, next step. If you've got all the resources at your disposal and the task is non-negotiable, but you still don't feel you're going to do a good enough job, can you have all those thoughts and feelings and still get the work done?

Yes, you can. You really can! So let's lean into that and run with it.

So what if your mind is telling you that Molly from marketing did a really good job on a similar project last week and there's no way you can compete with that? You're going to acknowledge that thought and unhook yourself from it: 'Oh, thanks, mind. But I'm not worried about that,' or: 'I'm having the thought that . . .', instead of fusing with it and identifying it as fact. It's just another unhelpful thought you can let go of. You've called it out and you're saying to yourself that you can do this in spite of those uncomfortable thoughts and feelings.

Another good technique is to break it down. If the project you're putting off feels too big and overwhelming, can you chop it up into smaller chunks? Doing it in twenty-minute segments with breaks in between might feel more manageable. Maybe you've got five sections of a report to write. Can you view each section as the assignment itself and snap yourself out of procrastination that way?

I'll tell you what I do, if you promise not to laugh. If I've got a piece of work I've really been avoiding, I like to make a big song and dance about it. I'll light some incense and put on frequency music for maximum zen. I get a lovely hot drink and change into the softest jumper I own – sensory stuff is really good, especially for highly sensitive people. I might even bring in the weighted blanket.

For me, it's about making the whole space as self-indulgent as possible while engaging as many senses as I can. OK, I'm not gonna lie, sometimes I get it all set up and I'm still like: 'Nope!' And so I just sit there and smell the incense.

Most of the time, though, it works. And yeah, joss sticks and meditation tunes might sound a bit woo-woo (OK, a lot woo-woo), but don't judge until you've tried it!

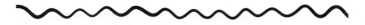

Ten ways to make sure you get shit done

1. Break it down by time or task

Putting the work into smaller, bite-size pieces makes it feel more doable, so see how many smaller tasks you can create from one big task and do those one by one. Or break it up by time and spend just five minutes on each task (you can tolerate five minutes), then, at the end, see if you can spend another five on it, and so on. You could even set a timer for a longer period of time – say, forty-five minutes – and plan to do only that much even if you feel you can do more.

2. Recognize your urge to procrastinate in a non-judgemental and non-blaming way

Maybe you feel a little uneasy or slightly worried, maybe there's some anxiety or a little frustration. If you make being aware of your urge to procrastinate a habit, then you will notice it before it gets too far and you can remind yourself that, in this moment, you have a choice to do something differently.

3. Worst first
Bang out the worst tasks first so all the tasks that remain feel easier.

4. Prep your environment
Make things easier for yourself and get rid of your phone or, at the very least, turn off the notifications. If you're sitting in an office with chatty colleagues, stick a pair of head-phones on so you're not tempted to join in their juicy convos. Figure out which parts of the day you feel at your opti-mum, your most productive or creative, and use this time to get started on your tasks every day. If you are consistent with this, now it's a habit, you're rewiring your brain and it becomes semi-automatic (gotta love neuroplasticity).

5. Nervous-system regulation
Use some of the exercises we've already discussed, such as grounding techniques like the 5–4–3–2–1 method we talked about in Chapter 2, breathwork, or vagal stimu-lation to activate the parasympathetic nervous system, and take yourself out of threat response, freeing up some headspace and getting your nervous system in the best condition to get started.

6. Tolerate your discomfort
Recognize any uncomfortable emotions or sensa-tions associated with doing the task and, instead of

procrastinating to avoid them, use it as an opportunity to practise tolerating it mindfully by observing it like a curious scientist without judgement, making space for it and letting it pass naturally.

7. Use your imagination

Why not use the power of your imagination for something good rather than it ushering you into catastrophic, negative images that keep you frozen? Instead of imagining failure, clearly visualize what it looks and feels like to complete the task. Savour that good feeling, notice where you can feel it in your body and use it to propel you into actually doing it.

8. Treat yo'self

It's very normal to end up feeling a little resentful about having to spend your time doing things you just don't wanna do when you could be doing something fun. Combat this by actively showing yourself how grateful you are for your efforts and rewarding yourself with something you do want to do so you a) don't get FOMO and b) positively reinforce getting shit done.

9. Find your compassionate voice

A compassionate voice is a wise one, so talk to yourself with love and kindness. Always. But be sure to look for any excuses you might be making to be OK with your procrastination and unhook yourself from them. My favourite excuse was: 'I don't have enough time now, so I might as well do it all tomorrow when I'm feeling fresh.'

10. Remove self-worth from the outcome

Your ability to achieve goals does not make you a good person, and vice versa. Disconnect that rule. You are already worthy because you are here, live and kicking.

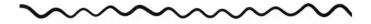

The culture of compare and despair

You know the colleague in your office who you compare yourself to? The girl with everything? She's newly promoted, popular, gets her work done to a consistently high standard, is always turned out immaculately in lovely clothes, not a hair out of place?

If her underlying core belief isn't great, then all those things you're seeing mean jack. In fact, they're in place to protect herself, and not being 'perfect' in any one of them will completely devastate her. She'll be working extremely hard to keep it up at the expense of her wellbeing. I work with high-functioning, well-put-together women who make it look easy. I was that person too!

It's not worth wasting energy stewing over comparisons to others when you really don't know what's going on behind the scenes.

Society is set up for comparison and competition. It's what creates hard-working people, and society thrives as a result. It makes sense from an evolutionary perspective, too. If we're the one acting wildly out of step in comparison to the rest of the group, we're going to get kicked out and, if we get kicked out, we're probably going to get eaten. Something is going to kill us. Therefore, it's in our interest to make sure we're doing enough (and we do this by seeing what others are doing) to keep us connected to the group.

So you can see that the idea behind comparison wasn't ever to make us feel defective – it was a natural, instinctive response, and it was key to our survival.

But the problem we have now, especially with social media, is that comparison is *encouraged*. You can see exactly how many people 'like' this person's picture compared to yours, and so now there's a 'best'. Someone will always be 'better'. And rather than being in small clusters, as we would have been thousands of years ago, we're now in huge groups with access to more and more people to compare ourselves to all the time, which heightens our already acute fears about being judged, rejected or not good enough.

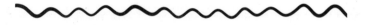

How to become more confident in your own abilities

- Refuse to negatively compare yourself to others; stay in your own lane.
- Face your fears and push through the anxiety to prove your inner critic wrong.
- Don't listen to your self-limiting beliefs.
- Identify your strongest points and where you could improve.

- Practise positive affirmations.
- Set small 'fearless' activities for yourself once a day.

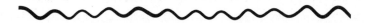

Using comparison as a force for good

Comparing doesn't always have to be a bad thing. If you're looking at the Instagram page of someone you admire and you're feeling inspired by them because you see a 'growth gap' (I got that phrase from Dr Melody Wilding, author of *Trust Yourself* – I love it), 'That's great!' Another person's ability to do something successfully does not take anything away from you, so let's see if you can use that feeling and try and get there too.

You might even message the person and say that you really appreciate what they're doing and you've been galvanized into action by it. Using social media to encourage people and to be positive and kind is much more meaningful than using it as distraction or a means of procrastination.

If, however, you are triggered by certain profiles, you have to delete those pages! I'm going to say it louder for those at the back: DELETE THEM!

+ ⁺ compare & being inspired by = GOOD ✚ ⁺
✱ comparing & despairing = NOT GOOD + ⁺

Weigh it up. Do an audit of all the accounts you're following across your social media regulars – TikTok, Instagram, Facebook, and so on. Have a scroll through your main feed and ask yourself what you get out of this page. Is it worth how you feel after you've seen it? If you're just left feeling rubbish, then it's going to serve no purpose other than to confirm your negative core beliefs, but we can stop this from continuing. Like, right now.

I have to be very boundaried around Instagram and selective about who I follow, because I know what I'm like. I once ended up with a £600 pair of shoes and I never go anywhere I could wear them. Like an idiot, I got caught up in the hype to nab them before they got snapped up, and I've worn them literally once. Basically, I'm ridiculously suggestible and, if I'm not careful, my bank account takes the hit. So, as a rule, I don't follow influencers who are trying to sell me clothes or shoes because, quite simply, I will buy them!

I follow other therapists because they give me new ways of thinking and, in this job, you never stop learning – there's new research out all the time and you need to stay on top of things.

I follow Beyoncé because she inspires me like no one else. I know she's a highly sensitive person (she didn't tell me this – I just feel it in my spirit, lol) and she's got a bit of anxiety, and yet she's still showing up and doing what she needs to do and being amazing at it, and that's what I love.

I follow my close friends and family, but even then, if it ever got to the point that what they were posting was making me feel bad, I would unfollow. I'm so strict with it because my boundaries around social media are about self-preservation. I don't have a personal Instagram, so if I'm scrolling through or commenting anywhere it needs to be about work.

I place a value on my time, and that's made it easier to put in and establish those limits. I don't want social media to cut into my work or relaxation time, so I remove all the distractions which are potentially going to put me in the mindset of doing things I don't want to do, aka googling how to lose 12 pounds in 6 days.

You can do all this too. Post pictures because you want to share your experiences with people, not because you want them to like your photo. This is a part of you that you're choosing to share with the people you're connected to on this platform. It doesn't matter if you don't get hundreds of likes; the value is in the connection.

We know that we can't stop the unhelpful thoughts coming into our minds. But we can choose what we do with them and, once you start to realize there's no use in comparing in this damaging way, the drive and impulse to do it will slow down.

Notice your thoughts and make the decision to redirect. You know what to do by now.

How to be perfectly imperfect

I want you to get to a point where you can accept that not everything in life will go perfectly. Sometimes you'll give a presentation and it'll be amazing; sometimes it'll be shit. Most of the time you'll be somewhere in the middle, and that's OK!

The thing is, I don't view the world through your negative core belief. I see it all much more objectively, because I can sit with the emotion and detach from the unhelpful thoughts (most of the time). It took some work to get to this point, but that's how I want you to end up seeing the world too, through this new, objective lens.

Once you have mastered mindfulness, then you'll be better at noticing when you're going down certain lines of thinking and being able to redirect your attention back to things you feel are important to you. It's very hard to do unless you actively practise those skills, though.

Try it my way. You've been doing it your way for so long. Let's not do any more of what is not working.

How to get over our fear of failure

Remember that you don't need to have all the answers, you don't need to pretend to be something you're not. It's OK if you're not a hundred per cent confident, it's OK if you're not a hundred per cent sure. You are still good enough; you can still move forward anyway.

remember that you DON'T need to have ALL the answers, you don't need to pretend to be something you're NOT.

Untangle yourself from other people's expectations, unhook yourself from the voice of those who criticized you as a child and made you feel unimportant or unloved, and tune into your voice that is so very full of love, compassion and pride for everything that you've conquered so far.

That's the only voice you need to listen to. That's the only validation you need.

When I see my clients connecting the dots and realizing they can go away and make the changes that will transform their lives, those are my eureka moments. I don't keep clients with me for any longer than they need to be – I am working to get people *out* of therapy. Not to sound harsh, but as soon as I can cut you loose, I will.

So I need you to see that you can do this by yourself. You are in control of your own behaviour, and that is the only way you're going to turn this around.

This is a process, and it's ongoing, but you can do it. Look back at all the times you thought you wouldn't be able to get through something, all the times you felt like giving up but didn't, all the times you came through for yourself. You did a whole pandemic! Even if you felt like you barely scraped through it. You are here. The evidence is stacking up that you can do hard things.

Be kind to yourself: you are capable, you deserve to feel worthy. And you have absolutely, fundamentally and unequivocally got this.

Now go and show the rest of the world just how brilliant you are.

no more excuses no more looking back

Start putting yourself FIRST for a change and just SEE what happens!

Closing Thoughts

Well, you made it through the book! How are you doing?

I hope that you're feeling more positive than when you started it. I hope you've got some clarity on why life might seem like such a struggle. And I hope you now know that it can be turned around.

Everything in this book has been tailored for you. Our experiences might be different, but we are all driven by the same underlying motivations. We want connections, we want security and we want to stay alive, so the ideas in this book apply to everyone, but especially to you who have picked it up.

Like I said at the beginning, don't let it gather dust. Keep on reading. After all, the reason I made it so pretty was so you would want to keep coming back to it.

It'll look super-cute on an easily accessible shelf, and you'll always know that there is the lovely book with the good stuff in it!

And remember, there are other people watching who might not have access to this book but will see you and your change and growth. You don't need to take on that responsibility, but just know that by healing and investing in yourself others will notice and think maybe they can do it too. You might even share your wisdom about how you got to this point, so you're not just helping yourself, you're helping the women around you because there will be plenty who look like they've got their shit together but have some kind of struggle going on behind closed doors.

You're not defective, you are human. If anyone had gone through the same experiences you have, they would act the same. Hopefully, by now, you've taken self-judgement off the table. Keep it off.

So this is it now: no more excuses, no more looking back. Start putting yourself first for a change and just see what happens.

And let me know! I can't wait to hear how you've kicked some ass and taken back control of your life and your happiness.

Acknowledgements

I'd like to thank my person, my family, my friends, my agent Sarah, Beth, and of course the team at Penguin for making this happen.